The Life-Changing 30-Day Health Plan

A Step-by-Step Guide to Changing Your Eating Habits and Achieving Lifelong Wellness

BY

Ladd Bagley

CONTENTS

INTRODUCTION

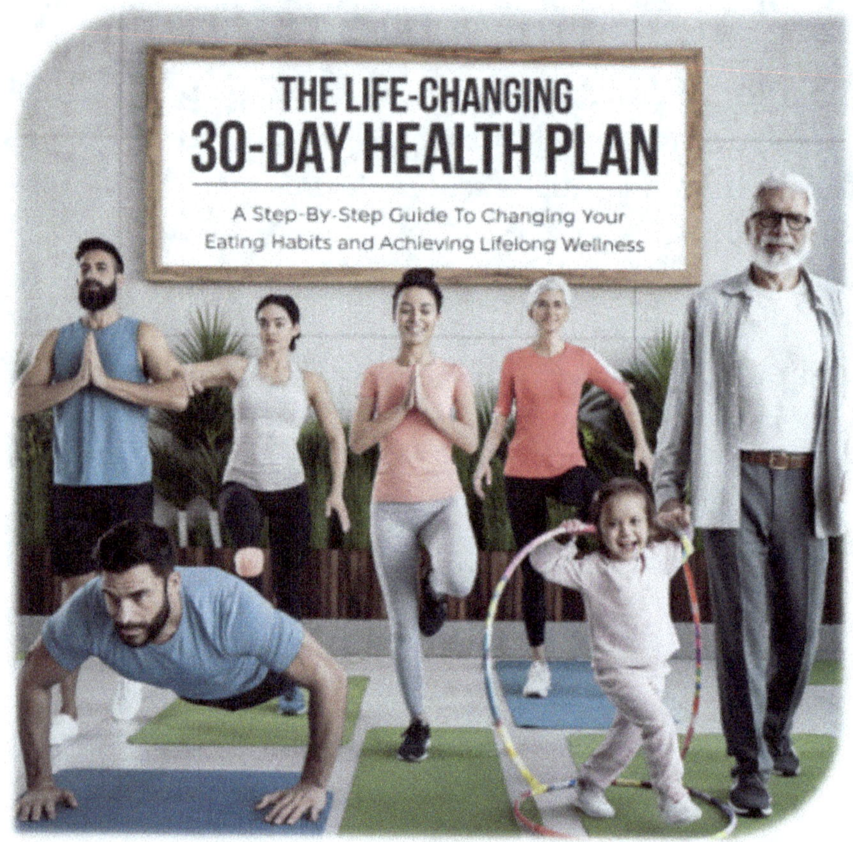

Our Journey to Health Starts Here

Welcome to "The Life-Changing 30-Day Health Plan," a transformative guide designed to help you take control of your health, reshape your habits, and set the foundation for lifelong wellness. In this journey, you'll learn how to overhaul not just your diet, but your mindset, physical activity, and lifestyle. Whether you're looking to shed some weight, gain more energy, or just feel better in your body and mind, this guide is structured to provide you with the tools, knowledge, and motivation you need to succeed.

Before we dive into the specifics of the plan, let's begin by addressing an important question: why 30 days? What makes a month-long commitment so powerful in changing your life?

Why 30 Days?

One of the key reasons this health plan focuses on a 30-day commitment is rooted in the science of habit formation. Studies show that it takes approximately 21 to 30 days to form new habits or break old ones. When you stick with a routine or behavior for this length of time, it becomes ingrained in your daily life. By consistently following the steps outlined in this guide for 30 days, you're not only giving your body the chance to adapt, but you're also rewiring your brain to support long-term positive behaviors.

The Science of Habit Formation

Our brains thrive on routine and repetition. The concept of neuroplasticity tells us that the brain can rewire itself based on repeated actions. When you consistently follow a new habit, neural pathways are strengthened, making the behavior easier to repeat without as much conscious effort. For example, if you start drinking a glass of water first thing every morning, after 30 days, it will feel automatic. This same principle applies to healthy eating, exercise, and mindfulness practices.

Breaking Bad Habits

In contrast, unhealthy habits, such as consuming too much sugar, skipping meals, or sitting for long periods, can also be broken during this 30-day window. By deliberately avoiding these negative behaviors and replacing them with positive ones, you can significantly reduce their grip on your life. The plan we've outlined isn't about crash diets or unrealistic restrictions—it's about creating a sustainable, healthy lifestyle that you can maintain well beyond these 30 days.

A Holistic Approach

This 30-day plan is different from other health programs because it takes a holistic approach. Too often, people focus solely on diet or exercise, neglecting other key aspects of wellness. Here, we emphasize not just nutrition, but also mindset, movement, and lifestyle. By addressing all of these components, you'll experience a more complete transformation that's not just physical, but also mental and emotional.

The Power of Mindset

Your mindset is crucial for success. This plan will help you develop a growth mindset, where you believe in your ability to change and improve. It's about adopting a positive attitude toward challenges, understanding that setbacks are part of the process, and seeing them as opportunities for growth rather than failures. We'll guide you through practices such as daily affirmations, visualization, and accountability to keep your mindset strong.

Movement and Exercise

Movement is an essential part of this journey. You don't need to spend hours in the gym, but you do need to incorporate daily activity to improve your overall health. This plan includes tips for getting started with exercise, how to stay consistent, and ways to enjoy moving your body. Whether you prefer yoga, walking, or strength training, there's a place for every kind of movement in this plan.

Lifestyle Adjustments

Lastly, lifestyle changes are crucial for long-term success. These include meal prepping, time management, stress reduction, and sleep optimization. By paying attention to how you live outside of the kitchen and gym, you'll create a well-rounded, sustainable approach to health that can fit seamlessly into your everyday life.

The 4 Pillars of Wellness

To simplify this process, we've broken it down into four main pillars: nutrition, hydration, exercise, and mindfulness. These pillars form the foundation of your health and wellness journey, and together, they will help you create a balanced, sustainable approach to feeling your best.

1. Nutrition

What you eat is the single most important factor in determining your health. Nutrition affects everything from your weight and energy levels to your immune system and mood. In this guide, you'll learn how to nourish your body with whole, nutrient-dense foods that fuel your metabolism and help you feel vibrant.

We'll break down meal plans, recipes, and tips for eating in a way that feels satisfying and sustainable. No extreme diets, no starvation—just simple, healthy eating habits that are easy to maintain.

2. Hydration

Water is the essence of life, and yet many people don't drink nearly enough of it. Staying properly hydrated is key to maintaining energy levels, supporting digestion, and even promoting clear skin. This plan will emphasize the importance of water and provide you with strategies for increasing your daily water intake.

We'll also discuss how to recognize the signs of dehydration and why certain drinks (like sugary sodas and excessive caffeine) should be minimized.

3. Exercise

Physical activity is about more than just burning calories—it's about improving your overall health, mood, and longevity. Regular exercise helps regulate blood sugar, boosts your metabolism, strengthens your heart, and promotes mental clarity. Whether you're a seasoned athlete or a beginner, this plan offers ways to integrate more movement into your life in a fun and sustainable way.

From strength training to cardiovascular workouts, we'll explore different forms of exercise and how to find what works best for you.

4. Mindfulness

Mindfulness isn't just about meditation—it's about being present and aware of your body, your feelings, and your environment. By practicing mindfulness, you'll develop a deeper connection to your food choices, your emotions, and even your fitness routine.

Throughout this guide, we'll incorporate mindfulness exercises that help you manage stress, improve your sleep, and stay present during your meals and workouts. This pillar is often overlooked in health plans, but it's a game changer in building lasting habits.

How to Use This Book

This guide is designed to be followed step by step, with each chapter building on the previous one. While you're welcome to read through it all at once, the best way to get the most out of this book is to treat it as a day-by-day guide for the next 30 days.

Follow the Plan in Sequence

The plan is structured to take you through the stages of transformation in a logical order. We begin by laying the groundwork—clearing out unhealthy habits, resetting your mind, and establishing a positive environment. Then, we focus on building momentum through smart eating and regular movement. Finally, we focus on sustainability, showing you how to maintain your results long after the 30 days are over.

Actionable Steps

Each chapter includes practical, actionable steps you can start implementing right away. From meal prepping tips to exercise routines, we've broken everything down into easy-to-follow instructions that make it simple to stay on track. No guesswork required—just follow the plan.

Checklists and Journal Prompts

Throughout the book, you'll find checklists, journal prompts, and reflection exercises to help you stay organized and connected to your progress. These tools are meant to keep you accountable and mindful of the changes you're making.

Adjust to Fit Your Life

While the book provides a structured plan, we also recognize that everyone's life and needs are different. You'll find guidance on how to customize the plan based on your individual goals, preferences, and schedule. Flexibility is key to creating lasting habits, so feel free to make the necessary adjustments while staying committed to the core principles.

Setting Realistic Expectations

Before we embark on this journey together, it's important to set realistic expectations. Transforming your health in 30 days is possible, but it's not about perfection or instant gratification. It's about progress and sustainable change. The goal is to lay the groundwork for healthy habits that will last a lifetime, not just quick-fix solutions that lead to short-term results.

Understanding the Process

Health is a marathon, not a sprint. Some days will feel easier than others, and there will likely be times when you feel like giving up. The key is to remain patient and consistent. The first week might be tough as your body adjusts to new habits, but by the end of 30 days, you'll be amazed at how far you've come.

Avoiding Perfectionism

Perfectionism is the enemy of progress. Expecting flawless execution every day sets you up for frustration and burnout. Instead, focus on doing your best each day, recognizing that every small step forward is progress. If you have a day where things don't go as planned, don't beat yourself up. Simply get back on track the next day.

Celebrating Small Wins

Don't wait until the end of the 30 days to celebrate your success. Along the way, you'll hit small milestones that are worth acknowledging. Whether it's drinking more water, resisting a sugary snack, or completing a workout, each victory counts and deserves to be celebrated.

Self-Assessment

Before diving into the program, it's essential to assess where you currently stand with your health habits and mindset. This self-assessment will help you identify areas where you can focus your energy and where you might need extra support during the plan.

Current Eating Habits

- How often do you eat processed or sugary foods?
- Are your meals balanced in terms of protein, healthy fats, and carbohydrates?
- Do you regularly consume fruits, vegetables, and whole grains?

Physical Activity

- How active are you on a daily basis?
- Do you have a consistent exercise routine?
- What types of movement do you enjoy, and how can you incorporate them more frequently?

Mindset and Stress Management

- How do you handle stress? Do you turn to food, alcohol, or other unhealthy habits?
- Do you have a positive mindset when it comes to your health and fitness goals?
- Are you ready to make changes, even if they feel challenging at first?

Sleep and Recovery

- Are you getting enough restful sleep each night?

- How do you feel when you wake up in the morning—energized or sluggish?
- Do you make time for rest and recovery, or are you constantly on the go?

By taking a close look at your current habits, you'll gain clarity on where you need to focus your efforts during the next 30 days. This honest self-reflection is the first step toward meaningful, lasting change.

Now that you've completed the introduction, you're ready to begin your 30-day health transformation. Keep this guide close, stay open to the process, and trust that you're capable of achieving the change you desire. Let's get started!

Part 1:
Building the
Foundation (Days 1-10)

Chapter 01

Mindset Matters – Setting Yourself Up for Success

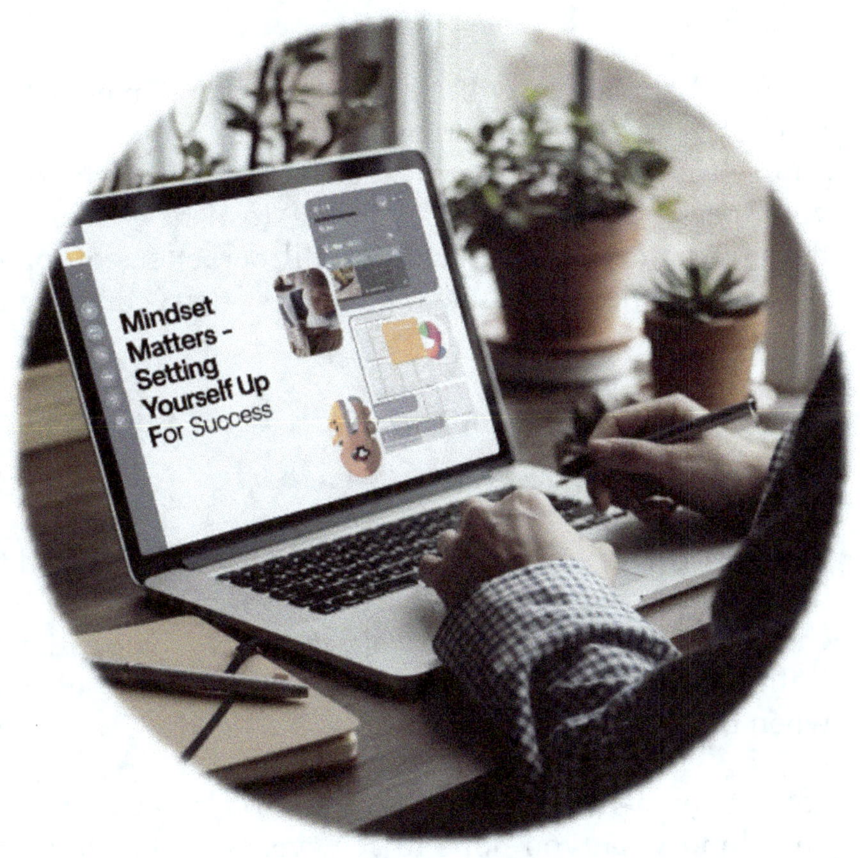

Embarking on a health transformation requires more than just meal planning and exercise routines. The most critical, yet often overlooked, component of lasting change is your mindset. Your thoughts, beliefs, and attitudes about yourself and your health can either propel you forward or hold you back. Success starts from within, and building a strong, positive mindset is the foundation for everything that follows in this 30-day journey.

In this chapter, we will explore the key elements that contribute to a growth-oriented mindset, so you can set yourself up for long-term success. By understanding your personal motivations, setting realistic goals, and developing mental resilience, you'll be better equipped to handle the inevitable challenges that come with change.

Understanding Your "Why" – Defining Your Personal Motivations for Change

Before you dive into any new health plan, it's essential to understand your "why." Why do you want to make this change? What are your deep, personal motivations? Without a strong sense of purpose, it's easy to lose focus when the going gets tough.

Take a moment to reflect on why you picked up this guide and what you hope to achieve. Is it to have more energy to keep up with your kids? To feel more confident in your body? To reduce your risk of chronic diseases? Everyone's "why" is different, but it needs to resonate with you on an emotional level. This emotional connection to your goal will fuel your determination when motivation wanes.

Action Step: Write Down Your "Why"

Grab a notebook or journal and write down your reasons for wanting to improve your health. Be specific and dig deep. For example, instead of writing, "I want to lose weight," expand it to something more personal: "I want to lose weight because I want to feel confident and strong in my body, and I want to be able to keep up with my family on our weekend hikes." Keep this statement where you can see it every day, as a reminder of why you started this journey.

Stay Focused on Your "Why"

Throughout this 30-day health plan, come back to your "why" whenever you face temptation or feel like giving up. Whether it's during a tough workout or when you're tempted by junk food, reminding yourself of your deeper purpose can give you the push you need to stay on track.

Visualization and Goal Setting – How to Set Realistic, Achievable Goals

Setting goals is essential to any health journey, but not all goals are created equal. Setting unrealistic, overly ambitious goals can lead to frustration and burnout, while vague goals can lack the clarity needed to spur action. The key to effective goal-setting is to be both specific and realistic.

SMART Goals

A great framework for setting health-related goals is the SMART method:

- **Specific**: Define exactly what you want to achieve.
- **Measurable**: Make sure your goal is quantifiable so you can track progress.
- **Achievable**: Ensure that your goal is realistic given your current lifestyle and time frame.
- **Relevant**: Your goal should align with your broader "why" and be meaningful to you.
- **Time-bound**: Set a deadline or time frame for achieving your goal.

For example, instead of saying, "I want to get in shape," a SMART goal might be: "I will go for a 30-minute walk four days a week for the next month to increase my activity level and improve my energy."

Action Step: Write Down Your SMART Goals

In your journal, write down one or two SMART goals for the next 30 days. Be specific, and make sure the goals feel challenging but doable. You don't want to overwhelm yourself by setting goals that are too far out of reach, but you also want to push yourself enough that you feel accomplished when you hit them.

Visualization: See Yourself Succeeding

Visualization is a powerful tool that top athletes, entrepreneurs, and successful people in all walks of life use to manifest their goals. The act of visualizing success can help you stay motivated and committed to the process.

Take a few minutes each day to close your eyes and imagine yourself achieving your health goals. Picture how it feels to be stronger, healthier, and more energized. Imagine yourself making healthy choices effortlessly, whether it's preparing a nourishing meal or completing a workout. This mental practice reinforces positive behaviors and primes your brain for success.

Creating a Positive Mindset – Tips for Overcoming Self-Doubt and Building Self-Confidence

Change isn't always easy, and you may face moments of self-doubt throughout this journey. The voice in your head might whisper, "I've failed before, what makes this time any different?" or "I'm too tired to work out today. It won't make a difference." These are limiting beliefs, and they can sabotage your progress if you let them take control.

How to Overcome Self-Doubt

The first step in overcoming self-doubt is recognizing when it creeps in. Pay attention to your internal dialogue—what are you telling yourself about your abilities? When you catch yourself thinking negatively, pause and challenge the thought.

For example, if you find yourself thinking, "I'm never going to reach my goal," reframe it into something positive, like, "I'm making progress every day, and each step brings me closer to my goal."

Building Self-Confidence

Self-confidence grows as you start seeing progress, but it also requires consistent reinforcement. Every time you make a healthy choice, congratulate yourself. Celebrate small wins along the way, whether it's completing a workout or resisting an unhealthy snack. These small victories add up and build your belief in your ability to succeed.

Action Step: Reframe Negative Thoughts

Keep a list of common self-doubting thoughts that tend to surface, and write down positive reframes next to them. For example:

- **Negative thought**: "I'll never be able to stick to this."
- **Positive reframe**: "I've made it this far, and I'm getting stronger every day."

Daily Affirmations – The Power of Positive Thinking

Positive affirmations are a simple yet powerful way to reinforce a healthy mindset. By repeating positive statements about yourself and your goals, you begin to believe them. Affirmations help you stay focused, motivated, and aligned with your long-term vision.

How to Use Affirmations

The best time to use affirmations is first thing in the morning, when your mind is fresh, or before challenging moments like a workout or meal prep. Write down a list of affirmations that resonate with you and repeat them out loud or in your mind each day.

Examples of daily affirmations for this 30-day health journey might include:

- "I am committed to making healthy choices that nourish my body and mind."
- "I am capable of achieving my goals, one step at a time."
- "I embrace progress, not perfection."
- "I am strong, healthy, and energized."

Action Step: Create Your Affirmations

Take a few minutes to write down 3-5 affirmations that reflect the mindset you want to cultivate. Keep these affirmations somewhere visible, such as on your bathroom mirror or phone background, and repeat them daily.

Accountability – Finding a Support System or Accountability Partner

Accountability is a crucial component of success, especially when it comes to health goals. Whether it's a friend, family member, or even a coach, having someone to check in with regularly can make a big difference in your motivation and consistency.

How to Find Accountability

Think about people in your life who are supportive of your health goals. It could be a partner, a friend, or even an online community. If you're comfortable, share your specific goals with them and ask if they'd be willing to check in with you periodically to see how you're progressing.

If you prefer a more structured approach, consider hiring a coach or joining a group fitness class where accountability is built into the program. Sometimes, simply knowing that someone else is paying attention to your progress can be enough to keep you going, even on days when your motivation wanes.

Action Step: Identify Your Accountability Partner

Write down the name of at least one person who will serve as your accountability partner. Reach out to them and explain your goals. Set up regular check-ins, whether it's weekly calls, texts, or even sharing progress on social media.

Preparing for Setbacks – Strategies to Handle Challenges and Slip-Ups

No journey is perfect, and setbacks are inevitable. You might skip a workout, indulge in a less-than-healthy meal, or feel overwhelmed by stress. What's important is how you respond to these moments, and whether you let them derail your progress or use them as learning experiences.

The Importance of Flexibility

One of the biggest pitfalls of any health plan is an "all or nothing" mentality. It's easy to think that one slip-up means you've failed and might as well give up. However, this black-and-white thinking leads to unnecessary guilt and frustration.

Instead, approach setbacks with flexibility and self-compassion. Understand that setbacks are a normal part of the process. When they happen, don't dwell on them—focus on the next positive choice you can make.

Action Step: Develop a Setback Recovery Plan

In your journal, write down a plan for how you will handle setbacks. For example, if you miss a workout, plan to go for a walk the next day. If you overindulge at a meal, focus on making your next meal healthy and balanced. Having a plan in place will help you respond with resilience rather than guilt.

Learning from Challenges

Every setback is an opportunity to learn and grow. Ask yourself, "What caused this setback? Was it stress, lack of preparation, or a lack of motivation?" Once you identify the root cause, you can adjust your approach moving forward. Maybe it means prepping meals ahead of time or scheduling workouts earlier in the day when you have more energy.

By focusing on your mindset from the start, you'll build the mental strength needed to stay consistent and resilient throughout your 30-day health plan. Remember, success starts with believing in yourself and staying connected to your "why." Each day is an opportunity to take one more step toward the healthy, vibrant life you envision.

With this solid mental foundation, you're ready to move forward and start taking action toward your goals!

Chapter 02

Mastering Your Kitchen – Pantry Cleanout & Food Prep

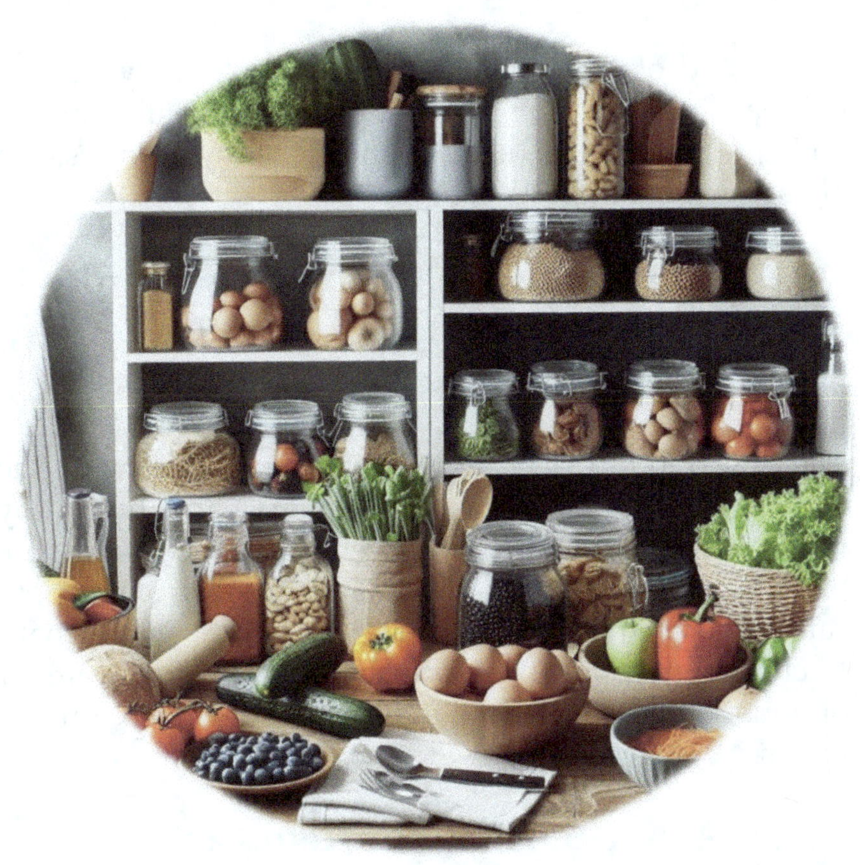

Your kitchen is the heart of your health transformation. It's where the choices you make every day begin. A well-organized, health-focused kitchen not only makes it easier to prepare nutritious meals but also helps reduce the temptation of grabbing something quick and unhealthy. In this chapter, you will learn how to declutter your pantry, stock it with essential healthy staples, and master meal prep strategies to set yourself up for long-term success.

By the end of this chapter, you'll know exactly how to overhaul your kitchen, save time with meal planning and prepping, and ensure that healthy choices are always at your fingertips.

Decluttering Your Pantry – How to Remove Processed, Sugary, and Unhealthy Foods

The first step in mastering your kitchen is removing the clutter—specifically, processed, sugary, and unhealthy foods that can sabotage your efforts. These foods are often high in refined sugars, unhealthy fats, and empty calories, which do little to support your health goals. Decluttering your pantry will make space for healthier options and reduce the temptation to fall back on old habits.

Action Step: Assess Your Pantry

Before you start tossing things out, take an inventory of your pantry. Pull out every item and evaluate whether it aligns with your new health goals. Ask yourself:

- Does this product contain a long list of unrecognizable ingredients?
- Is sugar or high-fructose corn syrup listed as one of the top ingredients?
- Does this food support my goals of clean, whole-food eating?

Foods to Toss

Here are common pantry items you'll want to consider removing:

- Sugary cereals and granolas
- Packaged snacks like chips, cookies, and candy
- Canned soups or sauces with high sodium and preservatives
- White bread, pasta, and other refined grains
- Soda, energy drinks, and sugary beverages

A Clean Slate

Once you've removed the unhealthy items, organize what's left. Group similar items together (e.g., grains, canned goods, spices) to make cooking easier. Use clear containers to store items like grains and nuts — this helps you see what you have and reduces waste. A tidy, organized pantry will inspire you to cook more and make healthier choices.

Stocking Your Kitchen for Success – Essential Healthy Staples

Now that your pantry is cleared of unhealthy foods, it's time to restock it with nourishing staples that support your 30-day health plan. A well-stocked pantry, fridge, and freezer will make it easier to whip up nutritious meals, even when you're short on time or creativity.

Pantry Essentials

Here's a list of healthy staples to keep in your pantry:

- **Whole Grains**: Quinoa, brown rice, oats, farro, and barley. These provide fiber and sustained energy.
- **Legumes**: Lentils, black beans, chickpeas, and kidney beans. Packed with protein and fiber, legumes are versatile and budget-friendly.
- **Nuts and Seeds**: Almonds, walnuts, chia seeds, flaxseeds, and sunflower seeds. These are great for snacking or adding to meals for a boost of healthy fats and protein.
- **Healthy Oils**: Extra-virgin olive oil, avocado oil, and coconut oil. Use these oils for cooking and salad dressings.
- **Spices and Herbs**: Cinnamon, turmeric, cumin, garlic powder, oregano, and basil. Spices add flavor without extra calories and are full of antioxidants.
- **Canned Goods**: Look for no-salt-added tomatoes, coconut milk, and low-sodium broths. These can help you create quick and flavorful meals.
- **Whole Grain Flours**: Almond flour, coconut flour, and whole wheat flour for healthier baking.

Fridge Staples

A well-stocked fridge is key to staying on track:

- **Fresh Vegetables**: Leafy greens, bell peppers, cucumbers, carrots, and broccoli. Keep a variety of colors to maximize nutrients.
- **Lean Proteins**: Chicken breast, turkey, grass-fed beef, and plant-based proteins like tofu or tempeh.
- **Eggs**: A versatile source of high-quality protein.
- **Plain Greek Yogurt**: Rich in probiotics and protein, perfect for breakfasts or snacks.
- **Fermented Foods**: Sauerkraut, kimchi, and pickles, which are great for gut health.

Freezer Staples

Frozen foods can be just as healthy as fresh if you know what to buy:

- **Frozen Vegetables**: Spinach, cauliflower, peas, and green beans are great for quick meals.
- **Frozen Berries**: Blueberries, strawberries, and raspberries are rich in antioxidants and perfect for smoothies or desserts.
- **Frozen Fish**: Wild-caught salmon, cod, and shrimp. These are quick to cook and provide heart-healthy omega-3 fatty acids.

Meal Prep 101 – Tips for Planning and Prepping Meals

One of the best strategies for staying on track with your health goals is meal prep. By preparing your meals in advance, you reduce the likelihood of making unhealthy food choices during busy or stressful times. Meal prep also saves you time during the week and helps you stick to portion-controlled, balanced meals.

Action Step: Create a Weekly Meal Plan

Start by planning your meals for the week. This doesn't have to be complicated—just focus on balanced meals that include protein, healthy fats, vegetables, and whole grains. You can either plan all three meals (breakfast, lunch, dinner) or start small by just prepping lunch or dinner.

For example:

- **Breakfast**: Overnight oats with chia seeds and berries
- **Lunch**: Quinoa salad with roasted vegetables and chickpeas
- **Dinner**: Grilled chicken with brown rice and steamed broccoli

Prepping Basics

Once you have your meal plan, make a grocery list based on the ingredients you'll need. Dedicate a couple of hours on the weekend to prep your meals for the week:

- Cook a large batch of grains like quinoa or brown rice.
- Roast a variety of vegetables like sweet potatoes, carrots, and broccoli.
- Grill or bake proteins such as chicken, turkey, or tofu.
- Portion out meals in containers for easy grab-and-go options.

Batch Cooking – How to Cook in Bulk

Batch cooking is a game-changer when it comes to saving time and ensuring you always have healthy meals on hand. By cooking large quantities of food at once, you can freeze meals for later, reducing the need to cook every day.

Benefits of Batch Cooking

- Saves time during the week by reducing daily cooking.
- Reduces food waste by using ingredients efficiently.
- Helps control portion sizes, making it easier to stick to your health goals.

Batch Cooking Ideas

Here are a few meal ideas that work well for batch cooking:

- **Soups and Stews**: Lentil soup, vegetable stew, and chili are easy to make in large batches and freeze well.
- **Casseroles**: Quinoa or brown rice-based casseroles with vegetables and protein can be made in large quantities and portioned out.
- **Grain Bowls**: Cook a big batch of grains (quinoa, farro, brown rice), then top with prepped vegetables, proteins, and a sauce.

Once your meals are cooked, portion them into freezer-safe containers. Label them with the date and meal name to stay organized. On busy days, simply defrost and reheat for a healthy, homemade meal.

Healthy Snack Ideas – Simple, Nutritious Snacks to Replace Unhealthy Choices

Snacking can either support or derail your health goals, depending on what you choose. Instead of reaching for chips or cookies, have healthy snacks on hand that satisfy your cravings and nourish your body.

Quick and Nutritious Snack Ideas

- **Hummus and Veggies**: Pair hummus with carrots, cucumbers, or bell pepper strips for a crunchy, fiber-rich snack.
- **Greek Yogurt with Berries**: A protein-packed snack that also satisfies your sweet tooth.
- **Nuts and Seeds**: Almonds, walnuts, or sunflower seeds are portable, filling, and full of healthy fats.
- **Apple with Almond Butter**: This combo provides fiber, protein, and healthy fats to keep you energized.
- **Hard-Boiled Eggs**: Prepare a batch of hard-boiled eggs at the beginning of the week for a quick grab-and-go protein snack.

Action Step: Stock Your Snack Drawer

Take a few minutes to prepare a snack drawer or box in your kitchen, fridge, or workspace. Fill it with healthy options like nuts, seeds, sliced veggies, and protein bars with clean ingredients. Having these snacks easily accessible will help you avoid the temptation of processed, sugary treats.

Tools for Success – Must-Have Kitchen Gadgets and Apps

Having the right tools in your kitchen can make healthy eating more enjoyable and efficient. You don't need a ton of gadgets, but a few key items can help streamline your cooking and meal prep.

Must-Have Kitchen Gadgets

- **Blender**: Perfect for smoothies, soups, and sauces. A high-speed blender can also blend nuts and seeds into healthy dressings or spreads.
- **Slow Cooker or Instant Pot**: Great for hands-off cooking. Use it to make soups, stews, and even grains with minimal effort.
- **Food Processor**: A versatile tool that can chop, slice, shred, and puree. Use it for everything from making hummus to shredding vegetables.
- **Glass Storage Containers**: Invest in a set of durable, leak-proof glass containers for meal prep. They keep food fresh and are microwave-safe.
- **Spiralizer**: Use this tool to turn veggies like zucchini and sweet potatoes into noodle shapes for low-carb, veggie-packed meals.

Helpful Apps

- **MyFitnessPal**: Track your meals, exercise, and progress with this user-friendly app.

- **Mealime**: Helps you plan meals, generate grocery lists, and provides simple recipes.
- **Yummly**: A recipe discovery app that allows you to filter recipes based on dietary preferences and restrictions.

By equipping your kitchen with the right tools and organizing your space for success, you'll make healthy eating an easier and more enjoyable part of your daily routine. When you have everything you need at your fingertips, it becomes much simpler to stick to your 30-day health plan and beyond.

Chapter 03

The First 10 Days – Resetting Your Body

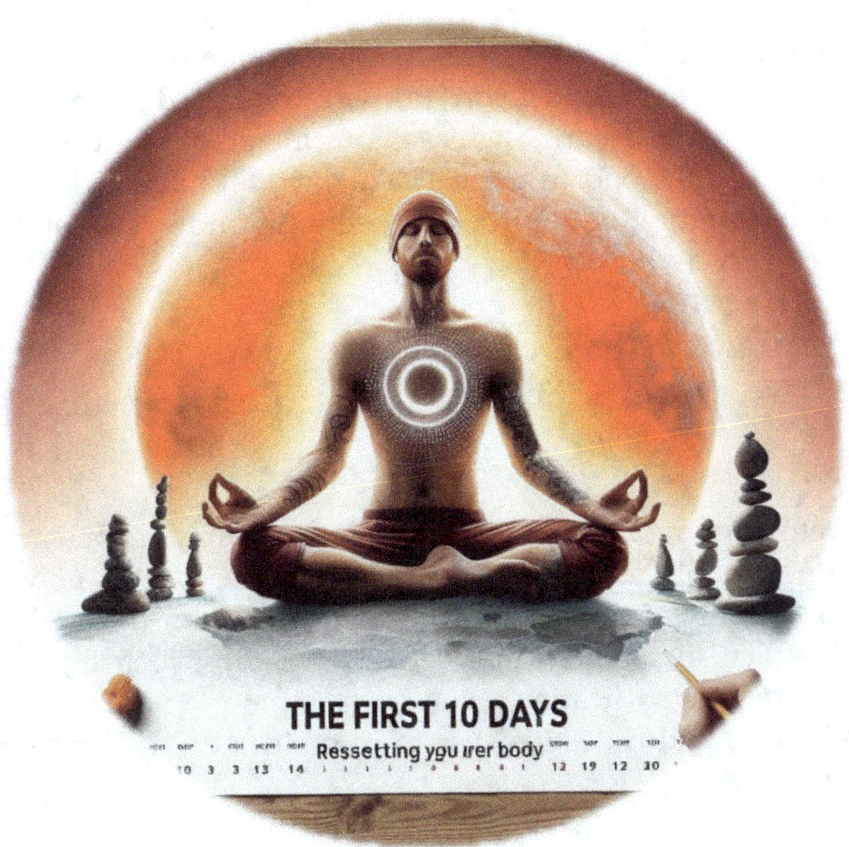

The first 10 days of your 30-day health plan are crucial for resetting your body and setting the stage for long-term success. During this initial phase, you will focus on cleansing your system, establishing healthy hydration habits, cutting out harmful foods, and rebalancing your nutrition. This period is about resetting your body's natural rhythms and setting a strong foundation for the weeks ahead.

In this chapter, you'll learn how to detox naturally through whole foods, stay properly hydrated, eliminate processed foods, and increase your intake of plant-based foods. By the end of these 10 days, you'll have a clearer understanding of your body's needs and how to nourish it effectively.

Starting with a Clean Slate – How to Detox Your Body Naturally Through Whole Foods

Detoxing your body doesn't require expensive supplements or extreme fasting. Instead, it's about eliminating toxins and resetting your system through a diet rich in whole, unprocessed foods. By focusing on natural detoxification, you can support your liver, kidneys, and digestive system in their natural cleansing processes.

The Basics of Natural Detox

Whole foods, such as fruits, vegetables, nuts, seeds, and whole grains, are packed with essential nutrients, fiber, and antioxidants that support your body's detoxification processes. These foods help to flush out toxins, improve digestion, and provide the vitamins and minerals needed for optimal health.

Key Points for a Natural Detox:

- **Increase Fiber Intake**: Fiber helps move waste through your digestive system and promotes regular bowel movements, which is essential for detoxification.
- **Opt for Organic Produce**: Whenever possible, choose organic fruits and vegetables to minimize exposure to pesticides and chemicals.
- **Focus on Hydration**: Proper hydration supports kidney function and helps flush toxins out of the body.
- **Limit Processed Foods**: Processed foods often contain additives, preservatives, and unhealthy fats that can hinder your body's natural detox processes.

Action Step: Clean Eating Plan

For the next 10 days, aim to eat a diet consisting primarily of whole foods. Create a meal plan that includes plenty of fruits and vegetables, lean proteins, and whole grains. Avoid processed foods, sugary snacks, and fried items. Focus on meals that are simple and nutrient-dense, such as:

- Breakfast: Smoothie with spinach, banana, berries, and chia seeds
- Lunch: Quinoa salad with mixed greens, chickpeas, cucumbers, and a lemon-tahini dressing

- Dinner: Baked salmon with roasted sweet potatoes and steamed broccoli

Hydration Habits – The Importance of Water and Tips for Ensuring You Stay Hydrated Throughout the Day

Staying hydrated is a fundamental aspect of overall health and plays a key role in your body's detoxification process. Water helps flush out toxins, maintain electrolyte balance, and support digestion and metabolism. Ensuring you're properly hydrated can also boost your energy levels and improve your skin's appearance.

How Much Water Do You Need?

A common recommendation is to drink eight 8-ounce glasses of water a day, known as the "8x8 rule." However, individual needs can vary based on factors like activity level, climate, and overall health. A good rule of thumb is to drink enough water so that your urine is light yellow in color.

Tips for Staying Hydrated

- **Carry a Reusable Water Bottle**: Keep a water bottle with you throughout the day as a reminder to drink regularly.
- **Infuse Your Water**: Add slices of lemon, cucumber, or berries to your water for a flavorful and refreshing twist.

- **Track Your Intake**: Use a hydration app or set reminders to help you meet your daily water intake goals.
- **Eat Hydrating Foods**: Incorporate water-rich foods into your diet, such as cucumbers, watermelon, oranges, and celery.

Action Step: Hydration Challenge

For the next 10 days, challenge yourself to drink at least 8 cups of water a day. Track your intake using a journal or app, and observe how increased hydration affects your energy levels and overall well-being.

Cutting Out Refined Sugars and Processed Foods – Why These Foods Are Harmful and How to Eliminate Them from Your Diet

Refined sugars and processed foods can have a detrimental impact on your health. They often lead to weight gain, increased cravings, and poor metabolic health. These foods are typically high in empty calories, unhealthy fats, and added sugars, which can contribute to inflammation and imbalanced blood sugar levels.

The Impact of Refined Sugars and Processed Foods

- **Refined Sugars**: Found in sodas, candies, baked goods, and many packaged snacks, refined sugars can cause rapid spikes in blood sugar levels, leading to increased cravings and energy crashes.

- **Processed Foods**: These foods often contain additives, preservatives, and unhealthy fats. They can be high in sodium and low in essential nutrients.

Strategies for Cutting Out Refined Sugars and Processed Foods

- **Read Labels**: Check ingredient lists for added sugars (e.g., high-fructose corn syrup, cane sugar) and avoid foods with a long list of unrecognizable ingredients.
- **Choose Whole Foods**: Focus on foods in their natural state, such as fresh fruits, vegetables, whole grains, and lean proteins.
- **Cook at Home**: Preparing your meals from scratch gives you control over ingredients and helps you avoid hidden sugars and unhealthy fats.
- **Find Healthy Substitutes**: Replace sugary snacks with healthier options like fruit, nuts, or yogurt.

Action Step: Sugar-Free Week

For the first 10 days, eliminate all sources of refined sugars from your diet. This includes cutting out sugary drinks, desserts, and snacks. Replace them with healthier alternatives such as fresh fruit, unsweetened yogurt, or a handful of nuts.

Increasing Plant-Based Foods – How to Incorporate More Fruits, Vegetables, and Plant-Based Proteins

Incorporating more plant-based foods into your diet is a powerful way to improve your health. Fruits, vegetables, legumes, and nuts provide essential nutrients, fiber, and antioxidants that support overall well-being and help to balance your diet.

Benefits of Plant-Based Foods

- **Nutrient Density**: Plant-based foods are rich in vitamins, minerals, and antioxidants that support various bodily functions.
- **Digestive Health**: High fiber content in fruits, vegetables, and legumes promotes healthy digestion and regularity.
- **Weight Management**: Plant-based foods are generally lower in calories and higher in nutrients, making them beneficial for maintaining a healthy weight.

Tips for Increasing Plant-Based Foods

- **Start Your Day with Fruits and Vegetables**: Add a serving of fruit or vegetables to your breakfast, such as spinach in your smoothie or berries with your oatmeal.
- **Experiment with Meat Alternatives**: Incorporate plant-based proteins like tofu, tempeh,

or lentils into your meals. These can be used in a variety of dishes as substitutes for meat.

- **Create Colorful Plates**: Aim to fill half your plate with vegetables at each meal. Choose a variety of colors to ensure a range of nutrients.

Action Step: Meatless Meals

For the next 10 days, include at least one plant-based meal per day. Experiment with recipes that feature legumes, tofu, or vegetables as the main ingredient. Track how you feel after incorporating more plant-based foods into your diet.

Balancing Macronutrients – Understanding the Role of Proteins, Fats, and Carbs in Your Diet and How to Balance Them

Balancing macronutrients—proteins, fats, and carbohydrates—is crucial for maintaining energy levels, supporting muscle growth, and regulating metabolism. Each macronutrient plays a distinct role in your body and contributes to overall health.

The Role of Each Macronutrient

- **Proteins**: Essential for muscle repair, immune function, and overall growth. Good sources include lean meats, fish, eggs, beans, and tofu.
- **Fats**: Provide energy, support cell function, and help absorb vitamins. Focus on healthy fats such as avocados, nuts, seeds, and olive oil.

- **Carbohydrates**: The body's primary source of energy. Choose complex carbs like whole grains, fruits, and vegetables over refined grains and sugars.

Tips for Balancing Macronutrients

- **Portion Control**: Use the plate method to balance your macronutrients. Fill half your plate with vegetables, one-quarter with lean protein, and one-quarter with whole grains or legumes.
- **Combine Foods**: Pair protein with complex carbs and healthy fats for balanced meals that keep you full and energized.
- **Monitor Your Intake**: Be mindful of portion sizes and aim to include a variety of macronutrients in each meal.

Action Step: Balanced Meals

For the next 10 days, aim to include all three macronutrients in every meal. Create a simple meal plan and track your daily intake to ensure you're meeting your balance goals. Adjust as needed based on your energy levels and hunger cues.

Listening to Your Body – How to Recognize Hunger, Fullness, and Energy Levels During the First Phase of the Plan

Being in tune with your body's signals is key to understanding how different foods and habits affect you. By paying attention to hunger, fullness, and energy levels, you can make adjustments to your diet and lifestyle that best support your health goals.

Recognizing Hunger and Fullness

- **Hunger**: True hunger is a physical sensation that comes from an empty stomach and is often accompanied by low energy. It's important to distinguish between physical hunger and emotional or habitual eating.
- **Fullness**: Eat slowly and pay attention to how your body feels. Stop eating when you're comfortably full, not stuffed. This helps prevent overeating and supports healthy digestion.

Monitoring Energy Levels

- **Pre-Meal**: Notice how you feel before meals. Are you feeling sluggish or energetic? Adjust your meals to address any dips in energy.
- **Post-Meal**: Pay attention to how you feel after eating. A balanced meal should leave you satisfied without causing fatigue or discomfort.

Action Step: Body Awareness Journal

Keep a journal for the first 10 days to track your hunger, fullness, and energy levels. Note what you eat, how you feel before and after meals, and any changes you experience. This will help you understand how your body responds to your new eating habits and make necessary adjustments.

By focusing on these key areas during the first 10 days, you'll set yourself up for success and create a strong foundation for the rest of your 30-day health plan. Remember, the goal is to make gradual, sustainable changes that will support your long-term health and well-being. Embrace this reset period as an opportunity to tune into your body's needs and make choices that align with your health goals.

Chapter 04

Smart Eating – Learning the Basics of Nutrition

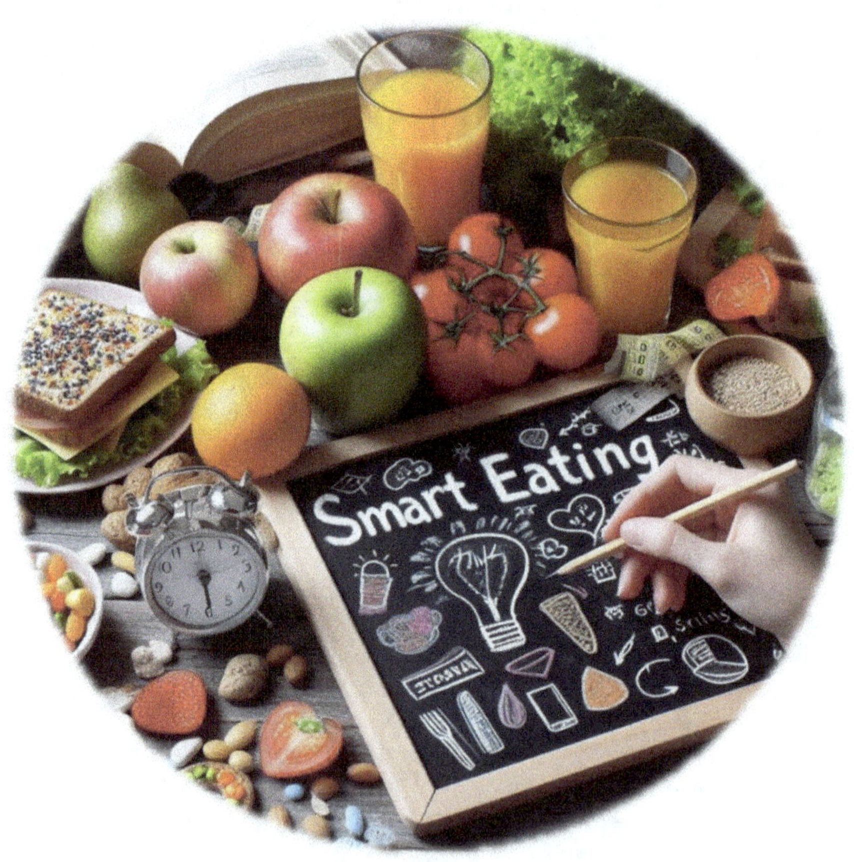

As you move into the second phase of your 30-day health plan, it's time to delve deeper into the fundamentals of nutrition. Understanding how to make smart food choices, control portion sizes, and incorporate nutritious ingredients will help you build momentum and sustain the positive changes you've started. This chapter focuses on the basics of nutrition, including nutrient density, portion control, reading food labels, and mindful eating. By mastering these principles, you'll be well-equipped to make informed decisions and continue your journey toward lifelong wellness.

Understanding Nutrient Density – The Concept of "Nutrient-Rich" vs. "Calorie-Rich" Foods

Nutrient density is a key concept in nutrition that helps you make choices that maximize the nutritional value of your food. Nutrient-dense foods provide a high amount of vitamins, minerals, and other beneficial nutrients relative to their calorie content. In contrast, calorie-rich foods often contain empty calories—calories that come from fats and sugars with little to no nutritional value.

What Makes a Food Nutrient-Dense?

- **Vitamins and Minerals**: Nutrient-dense foods are rich in essential vitamins and minerals that support various bodily functions. Examples include leafy greens, berries, and lean proteins.
- **Fiber and Protein**: High-fiber and high-protein foods contribute to satiety and support digestive

health. Foods like beans, lentils, and whole grains are great choices.

- **Low in Added Sugars and Unhealthy Fats**: Nutrient-dense foods typically have little to no added sugars or unhealthy fats. Focus on whole, unprocessed foods to keep your diet balanced and healthy.

Examples of Nutrient-Dense Foods

- **Fruits and Vegetables**: Leafy greens, bell peppers, berries, and sweet potatoes.
- **Whole Grains**: Quinoa, brown rice, oats, and barley.
- **Lean Proteins**: Chicken breast, fish, tofu, and legumes.
- **Healthy Fats**: Avocados, nuts, seeds, and olive oil.

Action Step: Nutrient-Dense Meal Planning

For the next 10 days, focus on including nutrient-dense foods in your meals. Create a meal plan that emphasizes fruits, vegetables, whole grains, and lean proteins. Avoid or minimize foods high in added sugars and unhealthy fats. Track how these changes affect your energy levels and overall well-being.

Portion Control – Simple Strategies to Avoid Overeating While Still Feeling Satisfied

Portion control is essential for managing your calorie intake and maintaining a healthy weight. Learning how to gauge appropriate portion sizes helps you enjoy your meals without overeating. This is particularly important as you progress in your health plan and aim to develop long-term, sustainable eating habits.

Techniques for Portion Control

- **Use Smaller Plates**: Eating from smaller plates can help you control portion sizes and prevent overeating. This visual trick makes portions look larger and more satisfying.
- **Measure Your Portions**: Use measuring cups or a food scale to familiarize yourself with standard portion sizes. This practice helps you become more aware of how much you're eating.
- **Practice Mindful Eating**: Slow down and savor each bite. Eating slowly gives your brain time to register fullness and helps prevent overeating.
- **Listen to Your Body**: Pay attention to hunger and fullness cues. Eat until you're satisfied but not overly full. Stop eating when you feel comfortably full.

Action Step: Portion Control Practice

For the next 10 days, practice portion control by using smaller plates and measuring your food. Note any changes in your eating habits and how it affects your hunger and satisfaction levels. Adjust portion sizes as needed to find what works best for you.

Reading Food Labels – What to Look for on Packaged Foods and How to Avoid Hidden Sugars and Unhealthy Fats

Understanding how to read food labels is crucial for making informed food choices. Food labels provide valuable information about the nutritional content of packaged foods, including calories, macronutrients, and ingredients. Learning to decipher these labels helps you avoid hidden sugars, unhealthy fats, and other additives.

Key Components of a Food Label

- **Serving Size**: Pay attention to the serving size to understand the nutritional information provided. Be mindful of how many servings you're consuming.
- **Calories**: Check the calorie content to ensure it aligns with your daily caloric needs. Remember that not all calories are created equal; focus on nutrient-dense options.
- **Nutrients**: Look for the amounts of protein, fiber, fat, and sugars. Aim for foods high in protein and fiber, and low in saturated fats and sugars.
- **Ingredients List**: Read the ingredients list to identify added sugars, unhealthy fats (e.g., hydrogenated oils), and other additives. Choose products with short ingredient lists and recognizable ingredients.

Common Hidden Sugars and Unhealthy Fats

- **Hidden Sugars**: High-fructose corn syrup, cane sugar, dextrose, and maltose are common sources of added sugars.
- **Unhealthy Fats**: Trans fats and partially hydrogenated oils are often found in processed foods and should be avoided.

Action Step: Food Label Analysis

For the next 10 days, practice reading food labels on packaged foods. Focus on identifying hidden sugars and unhealthy fats, and choose products with cleaner ingredient lists. Track any changes in how you feel and any improvements in your eating habits.

Healthy Substitutes – How to Replace Common Unhealthy Ingredients with Healthier Alternatives

Swapping out unhealthy ingredients for healthier alternatives is a practical way to improve your diet without sacrificing flavor or enjoyment. By making these substitutions, you can reduce your intake of harmful substances and increase the nutritional value of your meals.

Common Unhealthy Ingredients and Their Substitutes

- **Refined Sugar**: Replace with natural sweeteners like honey, maple syrup, or stevia. Use these in moderation to satisfy your sweet cravings.

- **White Flour**: Substitute with whole grain flours like whole wheat, almond, or coconut flour. These options provide more fiber and nutrients.
- **Butter**: Use healthier fats like avocado oil, olive oil, or coconut oil in place of butter. These fats provide beneficial nutrients and are less processed.
- **Cream and Heavy Sauces**: Replace with Greek yogurt, coconut milk, or homemade sauces made from blended vegetables. These alternatives are lower in fat and calories.

Tips for Successful Substitutions

- **Experiment with Recipes**: Try out new recipes that use healthy substitutes. This helps you discover tasty alternatives and integrate them into your regular meals.
- **Gradual Changes**: Start by making small substitutions and gradually incorporate more changes into your diet. This approach makes the transition easier and more sustainable.

Action Step: Ingredient Swap Challenge

For the next 10 days, focus on swapping out at least one unhealthy ingredient in your meals with a healthier alternative. Track the impact on taste, satisfaction, and overall health. Adjust your substitutions as needed based on your preferences and health goals.

The Power of Fiber – The Benefits of Fiber and How to Ensure You're Getting Enough in Your Daily Diet

Fiber is a crucial component of a healthy diet, offering numerous benefits for digestion, heart health, and weight management. Incorporating enough fiber into your daily diet helps maintain regular bowel movements, supports healthy blood sugar levels, and keeps you feeling full longer.

Benefits of Fiber

- **Digestive Health**: Fiber aids in digestion and helps prevent constipation by adding bulk to the stool and promoting regular bowel movements.
- **Satiety**: High-fiber foods take longer to digest, helping you feel full and satisfied for longer periods, which can aid in weight management.
- **Blood Sugar Control**: Fiber helps slow the absorption of sugar, reducing the risk of blood sugar spikes and crashes.

Sources of Fiber

- **Fruits and Vegetables**: Apples, pears, berries, carrots, and broccoli.
- **Whole Grains**: Oats, brown rice, quinoa, and barley.
- **Legumes**: Beans, lentils, chickpeas, and peas.
- **Nuts and Seeds**: Chia seeds, flaxseeds, and almonds.

Action Step: Fiber-Rich Meal Planning

For the next 10 days, plan your meals to include high-fiber foods. Aim to incorporate a variety of fruits, vegetables, whole grains, and legumes into your diet. Track your fiber intake and note any changes in digestion, satiety, and overall well-being.

Eating Mindfully – Tips for Slowing Down, Savoring Your Food, and Improving Digestion

Mindful eating is an approach that encourages you to be present during meals, focus on the sensory experience of eating, and listen to your body's hunger and fullness cues. Practicing mindful eating can improve digestion, enhance satisfaction, and promote a healthier relationship with food.

Principles of Mindful Eating

- **Slow Down**: Take your time to eat and savor each bite. Chew your food thoroughly and enjoy the flavors and textures.
- **Avoid Distractions**: Minimize distractions such as watching TV or scrolling through your phone while eating. Focus on your meal and the experience of eating.
- **Listen to Your Body**: Pay attention to hunger and fullness cues. Stop eating when you're comfortably full and avoid eating out of habit or boredom.

- **Appreciate Your Food**: Take a moment to appreciate the effort that went into preparing your meal and the nourishment it provides.

Benefits of Mindful Eating

- **Improved Digestion**: Eating slowly and mindfully helps improve digestion and nutrient absorption.
- **Increased Satisfaction**: Being present during meals enhances your enjoyment of food and can lead to greater satisfaction.
- **Better Portion Control**: Mindful eating helps you recognize when you're full, reducing the likelihood of overeating.

Action Step: Mindful Eating Practice

For the next 10 days, practice mindful eating by focusing on each meal. Set aside time to eat without distractions, chew slowly, and listen to your body's hunger and fullness cues. Reflect on how this practice affects your eating habits and overall satisfaction with meals.

By mastering these smart eating strategies during days 11-20, you'll build momentum and deepen your understanding of nutrition. This knowledge will empower you to make informed food choices, manage portion sizes, and cultivate a more mindful and satisfying eating experience. Embrace these principles as you continue your journey to health and well-being.

Chapter 05

Energizing Your Day – Revamping Your Daily Routine

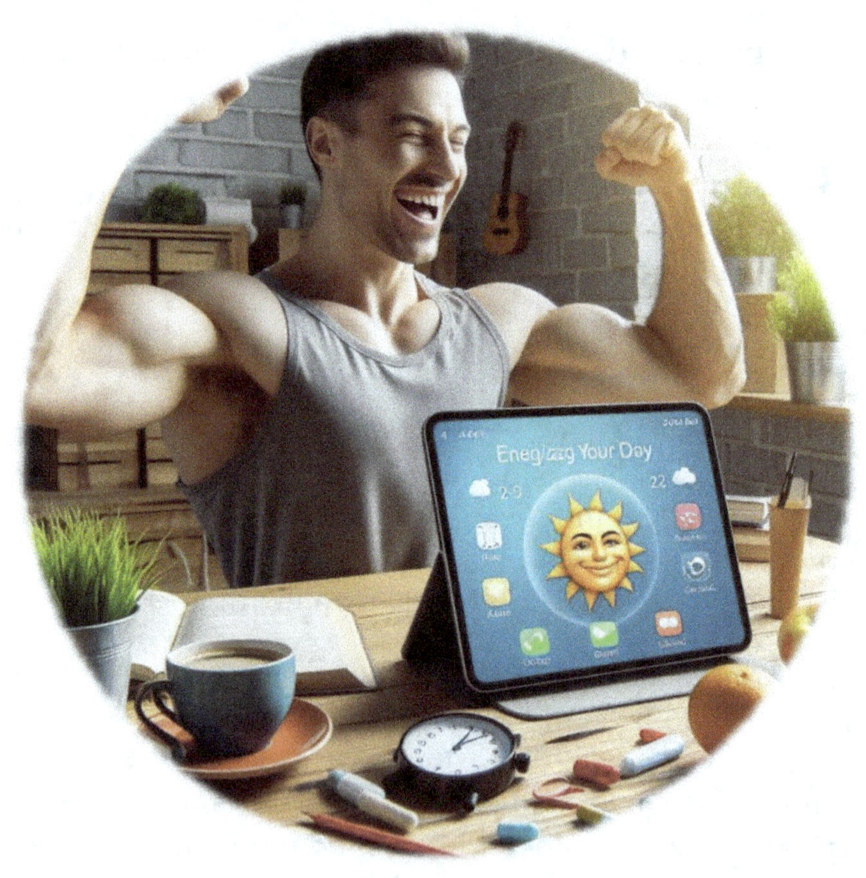

Revamping your daily routine to include energizing habits can significantly enhance your overall well-being and productivity. In this chapter, we will explore how to optimize your daily schedule for sustained energy, focus, and health. From the importance of a balanced breakfast to smart pre- and post-workout nutrition, we'll cover strategies to help you feel revitalized and maintain a healthy, energetic lifestyle throughout the day.

The Importance of Breakfast – Why Skipping Breakfast Can Harm Your Health and How to Make Quick, Healthy Meals

Breakfast is often touted as the most important meal of the day, and for good reason. A nutritious breakfast kick-starts your metabolism, provides essential nutrients, and sets the tone for your eating habits throughout the day.

Why Skipping Breakfast is Harmful

- **Metabolic Slowdown**: Skipping breakfast can lead to a slower metabolism, which may contribute to weight gain over time. Eating a balanced breakfast helps jump-start your metabolism and promotes healthy energy levels.

- **Energy Levels**: Breakfast provides the energy needed to start your day. Without it, you might experience fatigue, difficulty concentrating, and irritability.

- **Blood Sugar Regulation**: A morning meal helps stabilize blood sugar levels, reducing the likelihood of mid-morning energy crashes and unhealthy snacking.

Quick and Healthy Breakfast Ideas

- **Smoothie Bowl**: Blend fruits, vegetables, and a source of protein (e.g., Greek yogurt or protein powder) and top with granola, nuts, and seeds.
- **Overnight Oats**: Combine oats with milk or a dairy-free alternative, chia seeds, and your favorite fruits. Let it sit overnight in the fridge for a ready-to-eat breakfast.
- **Avocado Toast**: Spread mashed avocado on whole-grain toast and top with a poached egg, tomatoes, or a sprinkle of seeds.

Action Step: Breakfast Habit

Commit to eating breakfast every morning for the next 10 days. Experiment with different recipes to find what you enjoy most and what works best with your schedule.

Fueling Your Day with Balanced Meals – A Guide to Structuring Your Meals for Sustained Energy Throughout the Day

Structuring your meals to include a balance of macronutrients—proteins, fats, and carbohydrates—ensures that you have the energy to stay active and focused throughout the day. Balanced meals help maintain stable blood sugar levels and prevent energy crashes.

Components of a Balanced Meal

- **Proteins**: Essential for muscle repair and satiety. Include sources like chicken, tofu, fish, beans, or eggs.
- **Healthy Fats**: Support brain function and provide sustained energy. Opt for avocados, nuts, seeds, and olive oil.
- **Complex Carbohydrates**: Provide long-lasting energy. Choose whole grains, sweet potatoes, and legumes.

Meal Timing and Frequency

- **Three Main Meals**: Aim for three balanced meals each day—breakfast, lunch, and dinner. Ensure each meal contains a good mix of proteins, fats, and carbohydrates.
- **Snacks**: Include healthy snacks if you're hungry between meals. Opt for options like fruit, nuts, or yogurt to keep your energy levels stable.

Action Step: Meal Planning

Create a weekly meal plan that includes balanced meals and snacks. Focus on incorporating a variety of nutrient-dense foods and maintaining portion control. Track how these meals impact your energy levels and overall well-being.

Healthy Snacks on the Go – Portable, Nutritious Options That Keep You Energized Without Relying on Junk Food

Snacking can be a healthy part of your diet if you choose nutritious options that provide sustained energy. Portable snacks can help you avoid unhealthy choices when you're on the go.

Nutritious Snack Ideas

- **Fresh Fruit**: Apples, bananas, and berries are easy to carry and provide natural sweetness and fiber.
- **Nuts and Seeds**: Almonds, walnuts, and pumpkin seeds are great sources of healthy fats and protein.
- **Veggie Sticks with Hummus**: Carrot and celery sticks paired with hummus make for a satisfying and nutritious snack.
- **Greek Yogurt**: High in protein and calcium, Greek yogurt can be topped with fruit or nuts for added nutrition.

Tips for Smart Snacking

- **Portion Control**: Pre-portion snacks into small containers or bags to prevent overeating.
- **Plan Ahead**: Prepare snacks in advance to have healthy options readily available when you're busy.

Action Step: Snack Prep

Prepare a week's worth of healthy snacks and store them in convenient containers. Carry these snacks with you to avoid the temptation of unhealthy options.

Pre- and Post-Workout Nutrition – What to Eat Before and After Exercise to Maximize Your Energy and Recovery

Proper nutrition before and after workouts can significantly impact your performance, recovery, and overall fitness goals. Knowing what to eat can help you maximize your exercise benefits and reduce fatigue.

Pre-Workout Nutrition

- **Timing**: Eat a balanced snack or meal 1-2 hours before your workout. This helps fuel your exercise and maintain energy levels.
- **Focus on Carbohydrates and Protein**: Choose easily digestible carbs and a small amount of protein. Examples include a banana with a tablespoon of almond butter or a small smoothie with fruit and protein powder.

Post-Workout Nutrition

- **Timing**: Consume a post-workout meal or snack within 30-60 minutes after exercise to replenish energy stores and aid muscle recovery.
- **Combine Carbs and Protein**: Include both carbohydrates and protein in your post-workout meal. Good options are a protein shake with fruit or a chicken and quinoa salad.

Action Step: Workout Nutrition Plan

For the next 10 days, plan and prepare your pre- and post-workout meals and snacks. Adjust portions based on your exercise intensity and goals. Monitor how these adjustments impact your performance and recovery.

Incorporating Hydration into Your Day – How to Make Drinking Water a Habit Without Feeling Forced

Maintaining proper hydration is essential for energy levels, digestion, and overall health. Incorporating water into your daily routine can help you stay hydrated without feeling like a chore.

Tips for Staying Hydrated

- **Set Goals**: Aim to drink a specific amount of water each day (e.g., 8 cups). Use a water bottle with markings to track your intake.
- **Flavor Infusions**: Add natural flavors to your water with slices of lemon, cucumber, or berries to make drinking water more enjoyable.
- **Hydration Reminders**: Set reminders or use apps to prompt you to drink water throughout the day.

Action Step: Hydration Tracking

Track your water intake for the next 10 days and experiment with different flavor infusions. Evaluate how increased hydration affects your energy levels and overall health.

The Power of Sleep – Why Quality Sleep is Essential for Energy, Recovery, and Maintaining a Healthy Weight

Quality sleep is a critical component of overall health and well-being. Adequate rest supports energy levels, recovery, and weight management, making it an essential part of your daily routine.

Benefits of Quality Sleep

- **Energy and Cognitive Function**: Good sleep enhances energy levels, concentration, and memory.
- **Muscle Recovery**: During deep sleep, your body repairs and builds muscle, which is important for fitness and recovery.
- **Weight Management**: Poor sleep can disrupt hormones that regulate hunger, leading to increased appetite and potential weight gain.

Tips for Improving Sleep Quality

- **Establish a Routine**: Go to bed and wake up at the same time each day to regulate your body's internal clock.
- **Create a Relaxing Environment**: Keep your bedroom cool, dark, and quiet. Consider using a white noise machine or blackout curtains if needed.
- **Limit Stimulants**: Avoid caffeine and heavy meals close to bedtime. Instead, engage in relaxing activities such as reading or taking a warm bath.

Action Step: Sleep Improvement Plan

For the next 10 days, focus on improving your sleep quality by establishing a consistent sleep schedule and creating a relaxing bedtime routine. Track any changes in your energy levels and overall health.

By incorporating these strategies into your daily routine during days 11-20, you'll enhance your energy levels, improve your focus, and support your overall well-being. Revamping your routine to include balanced meals, healthy snacks, proper hydration, and quality sleep will help you build lasting habits and sustain your progress throughout your 30-day health plan.

Part 2: Building Momentum (Days 11-20)

Chapter 06

Physical Activity – Moving with Purpose

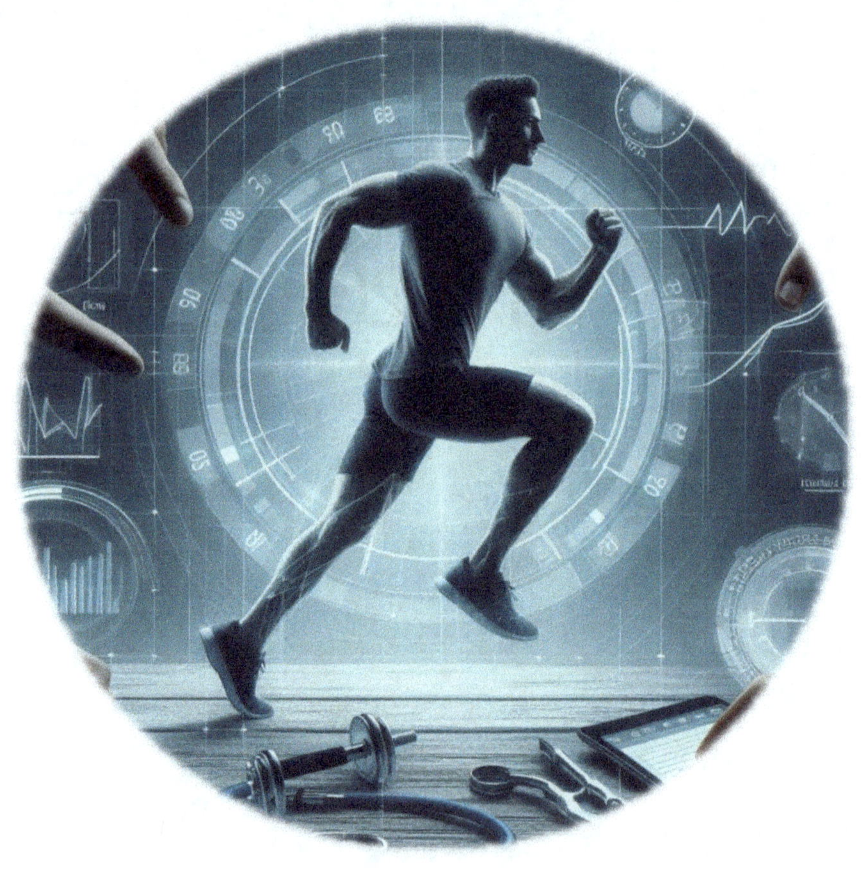

Incorporating physical activity into your daily routine is crucial for overall health and well-being. This chapter will guide you through selecting the right exercise routine, understanding the benefits of different types of workouts, and finding ways to stay active throughout the day. By moving with purpose and integrating exercise into your lifestyle, you'll enhance your fitness, improve your mood, and support your long-term health goals.

Finding Your Fitness Groove – How to Choose an Exercise Routine That Fits Your Lifestyle and Goals

Choosing the right exercise routine is essential for maintaining motivation and achieving your fitness goals. The key is to find activities that you enjoy and that align with your lifestyle and objectives.

Assess Your Fitness Goals

- **Weight Loss**: If your primary goal is weight loss, consider incorporating a mix of cardio and strength training. Cardio helps burn calories, while strength training builds muscle and boosts metabolism.
- **Muscle Building**: For muscle growth, focus on strength training exercises such as weight lifting, resistance bands, or bodyweight exercises.
- **General Fitness**: If you're aiming for overall fitness, a combination of cardio, strength training, and flexibility exercises will provide balanced benefits.

Identify Your Preferences

- **Solo vs. Group Workouts**: Decide if you prefer working out alone or in a group setting. Group classes can provide motivation and social interaction, while solo workouts offer flexibility and independence.
- **Indoor vs. Outdoor Activities**: Choose between indoor activities (e.g., gym workouts, yoga) and outdoor exercises (e.g., running, hiking) based on your preferences and weather conditions.

Create a Balanced Routine

- **Frequency**: Aim for at least 150 minutes of moderate-intensity cardio or 75 minutes of vigorous-intensity cardio per week, combined with two or more days of strength training.
- **Variety**: Include a mix of different exercises to prevent boredom and target various muscle groups. This can include cardio, strength training, flexibility exercises, and recreational activities.

Action Step: Fitness Assessment

Conduct a fitness assessment to determine your current fitness level and goals. Create a weekly exercise plan that incorporates a variety of activities and aligns with your preferences and objectives.

The Benefits of Strength Training – Why Building Muscle is Key to Metabolism and Overall Health

Strength training is an essential component of a well-rounded fitness routine. Building muscle through resistance exercises offers numerous benefits beyond just increasing strength.

Benefits of Strength Training

- **Increased Metabolism**: Muscle tissue burns more calories at rest compared to fat tissue. Building muscle helps boost your metabolism and supports weight management.
- **Improved Bone Health**: Strength training increases bone density, reducing the risk of osteoporosis and fractures.
- **Enhanced Functional Fitness**: Strong muscles improve your ability to perform daily activities and reduce the risk of injuries.

Types of Strength Training

- **Free Weights**: Use dumbbells, barbells, or kettlebells to perform a variety of exercises targeting different muscle groups.
- **Bodyweight Exercises**: Incorporate exercises like push-ups, squats, and lunges that use your own body weight as resistance.
- **Resistance Bands**: Use bands to add resistance to your workouts and target specific muscle groups.

Creating a Strength Training Routine

- **Reps and Sets**: Aim for 8-12 repetitions per set, with 2-3 sets per exercise. Adjust the weight or resistance based on your fitness level.
- **Rest and Recovery**: Allow at least 48 hours of rest between strength training sessions for the same muscle group to promote recovery and prevent overtraining.

Action Step: Strength Training Plan

Develop a strength training plan that includes exercises targeting major muscle groups. Aim to incorporate strength training into your routine 2-3 times per week and track your progress over time.

Incorporating Cardio for Heart Health – Simple Ways to Add Heart-Healthy Cardio into Your Routine

Cardiovascular exercise, or cardio, is crucial for maintaining heart health and overall fitness. Incorporating cardio into your routine can improve your cardiovascular system, boost your energy levels, and support weight management.

Benefits of Cardio

- **Heart Health**: Regular cardio exercise strengthens the heart, improves circulation, and reduces the risk of heart disease.
- **Increased Endurance**: Cardio workouts improve your stamina and ability to perform daily activities with less fatigue.

- **Calorie Burn**: Cardio exercises help burn calories and support weight loss or maintenance.

Types of Cardio Workouts

- **Walking or Jogging**: Simple and accessible forms of cardio that can be done outdoors or on a treadmill.
- **Cycling**: A low-impact cardio option that can be performed on a stationary bike or outdoors.
- **Swimming**: Provides a full-body workout and is gentle on the joints, making it suitable for people with joint issues.
- **High-Intensity Interval Training (HIIT)**: Alternates between periods of intense exercise and rest, offering an effective and time-efficient cardio workout.

Incorporating Cardio into Your Routine

- **Frequency**: Aim for at least 150 minutes of moderate-intensity cardio or 75 minutes of vigorous-intensity cardio per week.
- **Variety**: Mix different types of cardio exercises to prevent boredom and target different aspects of fitness.

Action Step: Cardio Integration

Add at least three cardio sessions to your weekly exercise routine. Experiment with different types of cardio to find what you enjoy most and track your improvements in endurance and overall fitness.

Everyday Movement Matters – How to Stay Active Throughout the Day Even if You Can't Get to the Gym

Incorporating movement into your daily routine, even when you can't make it to the gym, is essential for maintaining overall health and fitness. Small changes throughout the day can add up and contribute to your overall activity levels.

Tips for Staying Active

- **Take the Stairs**: Opt for stairs instead of elevators or escalators whenever possible.
- **Walk or Bike**: Use walking or biking as a mode of transportation for short trips or errands.
- **Standing Desk**: Consider using a standing desk or an adjustable workstation to reduce sedentary time.
- **Short Activity Breaks**: Incorporate short activity breaks during your workday. Perform quick exercises or stretches to keep your body moving.

Benefits of Everyday Movement

- **Increased Energy**: Regular movement throughout the day can help combat fatigue and boost energy levels.
- **Improved Posture**: Staying active helps maintain good posture and reduces the risk of back and neck pain.

- **Enhanced Mental Health**: Movement throughout the day can improve mood and reduce stress.

Action Step: Daily Movement Goals

Set daily movement goals and incorporate small activities into your routine. Track your progress and adjust your goals as needed to ensure you stay active throughout the day.

Stretching and Mobility – The Importance of Flexibility and How to Incorporate Daily Stretching

Flexibility and mobility are essential components of a well-rounded fitness routine. Regular stretching and mobility exercises improve range of motion, reduce the risk of injury, and enhance overall movement quality.

Benefits of Stretching and Mobility

- **Improved Flexibility**: Regular stretching increases flexibility, which can enhance performance in other exercises and daily activities.
- **Reduced Muscle Tension**: Stretching helps relieve muscle tension and prevent stiffness.
- **Enhanced Recovery**: Incorporating stretching into your routine can aid in muscle recovery and reduce soreness after workouts.

Types of Stretching

- **Static Stretching**: Involves holding a stretch for 15-60 seconds to improve flexibility. Perform static stretches after workouts or as a separate routine.
- **Dynamic Stretching**: Involves moving parts of your body through their full range of motion. Use dynamic stretching as part of your warm-up routine before exercise.
- **Foam Rolling**: Use a foam roller to perform self-myofascial release, which helps release muscle tightness and improve mobility.

Incorporating Stretching into Your Routine

- **Daily Routine**: Dedicate 5-10 minutes each day to stretching and mobility exercises. Focus on major muscle groups and areas of tension.
- **Post-Workout**: Incorporate static stretching after workouts to help cool down and improve flexibility.

Action Step: Stretching Routine

Develop a daily stretching routine that includes a mix of static and dynamic stretches. Incorporate foam rolling and mobility exercises to enhance overall flexibility and movement quality.

Exercise and Mood – How Regular Physical Activity Can Improve Your Mental Health and Well-Being

Regular physical activity has profound effects on mental health and emotional well-being. Exercise can help reduce stress, improve mood, and enhance overall quality of life.

Benefits of Exercise on Mental Health

- **Mood Enhancement**: Exercise stimulates the release of endorphins, which are natural mood lifters. Regular physical activity can help reduce symptoms of depression and anxiety.
- **Stress Reduction**: Exercise helps lower cortisol levels, reducing stress and promoting relaxation.
- **Improved Sleep**: Regular exercise can improve sleep quality and help manage insomnia or other sleep-related issues.

Incorporating Exercise for Mental Health

- **Find Activities You Enjoy**: Choose exercises that you find enjoyable and rewarding. This will make it easier to stay consistent and reap the mental health benefits.
- **Set Realistic Goals**: Establish achievable fitness goals that align with your mental health objectives. Celebrate your progress and stay motivated.

Action Step: Mental Health and Exercise Integration

Incorporate physical activity into your routine with the goal of improving your mental health. Track changes in mood and stress levels as you engage in regular exercise and adjust your routine based on your findings.

By focusing on these key aspects of physical activity during days 11-20, you'll build a solid foundation for incorporating exercise into your daily routine. Choosing the right activities, understanding the benefits of different types of workouts, and staying active throughout the day will support your fitness goals and enhance your overall well-being. Embrace these principles as you continue your journey to health and vitality.

Chapter 07

Overcoming Plateaus –
Breaking Through the Mid-
Program Slump

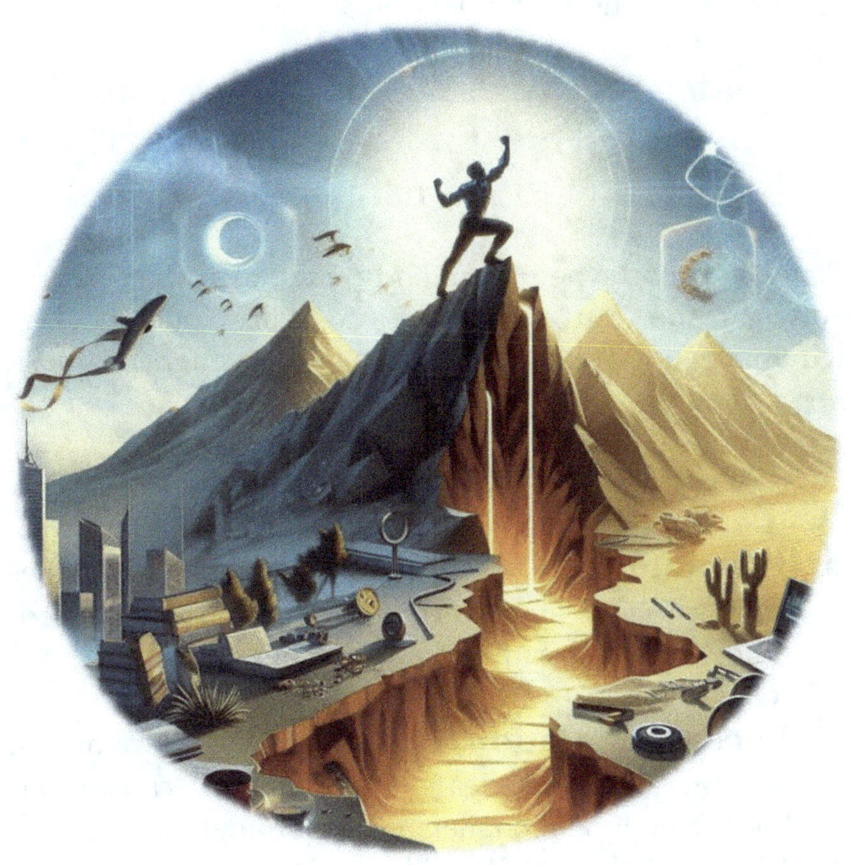

As you approach the final stretch of your 30-day health plan, you may encounter a plateau—a period where progress seems to stall despite your continued efforts. Plateaus can be frustrating, but they are a normal part of any transformative journey. This chapter will guide you through understanding plateaus, tracking your progress effectively, and making necessary adjustments to break through this mid-program slump. By staying focused and adaptable, you can continue to move forward and achieve your long-term goals.

Understanding Plateaus – Why They Happen and How to Break Through Them with Adjustments

Plateaus occur when your body adapts to the changes you've made, causing progress to stall. Understanding why plateaus happen and how to address them is crucial for continuing your progress.

Why Plateaus Happen

- **Adaptation**: As you progress, your body becomes more efficient at performing the same exercises or following the same diet, leading to diminished returns.
- **Lack of Variation**: Repeating the same workout or eating plan can lead to a plateau because your body is no longer challenged or stimulated.
- **Overtraining or Under-recovery**: Not allowing sufficient time for rest and recovery can hinder progress and contribute to plateaus.

Breaking Through Plateaus

- **Increase Intensity**: Make your workouts more challenging by increasing the weight, speed, or duration of your exercises.
- **Change Your Routine**: Introduce new exercises or activities to stimulate different muscle groups and prevent adaptation.
- **Adjust Your Diet**: Modify your macronutrient ratios or meal timing to address changes in your metabolism and energy needs.

Action Step: Plateau Assessment

Identify any plateaus in your progress and evaluate potential causes. Implement changes to your routine or diet and monitor their impact on your progress over the next week.

Tracking Your Progress – How to Measure Success Without Relying Solely on the Scale

While the scale is a common tool for measuring progress, it doesn't provide a complete picture of your health and fitness journey. Incorporating other methods to track your progress can offer a more comprehensive view.

Alternative Progress Indicators

- **Body Measurements**: Track changes in measurements such as waist, hips, and arms to monitor shifts in body composition.

- **Fitness Levels**: Record improvements in strength, endurance, and flexibility. For example, note how much weight you can lift or how long you can run.
- **Energy and Mood**: Evaluate how your energy levels and mood have changed. Enhanced energy and mood improvements are significant indicators of progress.
- **Clothing Fit**: Pay attention to how your clothes fit and feel. Looser-fitting clothes can signal changes in body composition.

Setting Up a Tracking System

- **Journaling**: Keep a fitness journal to record workouts, dietary changes, and personal reflections. This helps you track patterns and identify areas for improvement.
- **Photos**: Take progress photos from multiple angles in consistent lighting to visually track changes over time.

Action Step: Comprehensive Tracking

Utilize multiple methods to track your progress beyond the scale. Assess changes in body measurements, fitness levels, energy, and mood over the next 10 days and adjust your strategies accordingly.

Tweaking Your Diet – Small Adjustments to Macronutrients and Meal Timing That Can Reignite Progress

Adjusting your diet can help break through a plateau by addressing changes in your metabolism and energy needs. Small tweaks can reignite progress and support continued success.

Adjusting Macronutrients

- **Protein**: Increase protein intake to support muscle repair and growth. Incorporate lean protein sources such as chicken, fish, tofu, or legumes.
- **Carbohydrates**: Evaluate your carbohydrate intake and adjust based on your activity level. Opt for complex carbohydrates like whole grains and vegetables.
- **Fats**: Ensure you're consuming healthy fats from sources like avocados, nuts, and olive oil. Avoid excessive intake of unhealthy fats.

Meal Timing

- **Pre- and Post-Workout Nutrition**: Ensure you're consuming balanced meals or snacks before and after workouts to optimize performance and recovery.
- **Meal Frequency**: Consider adjusting the frequency of your meals and snacks to better align with your energy needs and hunger cues.

Action Step: Dietary Adjustment Plan

Review your current diet and identify areas for potential adjustments. Make small changes to macronutrient ratios or meal timing and observe their impact on your progress over the next week.

Varying Your Workouts – How Changing Your Fitness Routine Can Boost Both Results and Motivation

Introducing variety into your fitness routine can help break through plateaus, prevent boredom, and keep you motivated. Changing your workouts can challenge your body in new ways and enhance your results.

Benefits of Workout Variation

- **Prevents Adaptation**: New exercises or routines prevent your body from adapting, ensuring continued progress.
- **Reduces Boredom**: Variety keeps workouts interesting and enjoyable, increasing adherence to your fitness plan.
- **Targets Different Muscle Groups**: Different exercises work various muscle groups, leading to more balanced strength and fitness.

Strategies for Varying Your Workouts

- **Change Exercises**: Swap out familiar exercises for new ones that target the same muscle groups.
- **Alter Intensity**: Adjust the intensity of your workouts by changing weights, resistance, or speed.

- **Try New Activities**: Incorporate different forms of exercise such as swimming, cycling, or group fitness classes.

Action Step: Workout Variation Plan

Create a plan to introduce variety into your workouts. Experiment with new exercises or activities and track their impact on your progress and motivation.

Staying Mentally Strong – Dealing with Frustration and Keeping Your Focus on the Bigger Picture

Maintaining mental strength and focus is crucial for overcoming plateaus and staying committed to your health goals. Developing resilience and a positive mindset will help you navigate challenges and continue making progress.

Strategies for Mental Strength

- **Set Realistic Expectations**: Understand that plateaus are a normal part of the process and not a reflection of failure.
- **Practice Self-Compassion**: Be kind to yourself and avoid negative self-talk. Recognize your efforts and celebrate your achievements.
- **Stay Focused on Your Goals**: Remind yourself of your long-term goals and the reasons why you started your health journey.

Coping with Frustration

- **Mindfulness and Meditation**: Engage in mindfulness practices or meditation to manage stress and maintain a positive outlook.
- **Seek Support**: Reach out to friends, family, or a support group for encouragement and motivation during challenging times.

Action Step: Mental Resilience Plan

Develop strategies to maintain mental strength and focus throughout your journey. Incorporate mindfulness practices, positive affirmations, and support systems into your routine.

Reassessing Your Goals – Checking In on Your Progress and Making Sure Your Goals Still Align with Your Vision

As you approach the final days of your 30-day plan, it's essential to reassess your goals and ensure they still align with your vision. Evaluating your progress and adjusting your goals will help you stay on track and plan for long-term success.

Evaluating Your Progress

- **Review Achievements**: Reflect on the progress you've made towards your goals. Assess changes in fitness, nutrition, and overall health.
- **Identify Areas for Improvement**: Determine any areas where you may need additional focus or adjustments. Consider whether your current goals still align with your evolving needs and aspirations.

Setting Long-Term Goals

- **Adjust Goals**: Based on your progress and reassessment, modify your long-term goals to reflect your current achievements and future aspirations.
- **Create a Plan**: Develop a plan to maintain and build on your progress. Set new milestones and action steps to continue your journey towards lifelong wellness.

Action Step: Goal Reassessment

Reassess your goals and progress over the next week. Adjust your goals as needed and create a plan to continue your health journey beyond the 30-day program.

By addressing plateaus, tracking progress comprehensively, and making necessary adjustments during days 21-30, you'll be better equipped to overcome challenges and achieve lasting success. Embrace these strategies to break through the mid-program slump, stay mentally strong, and set yourself up for long-term health and well-being.

Part 3: Transformation and Long-Term Success (Days 21-30)

Chapter 08

Fine-Tuning Your Nutrition –
Advanced Strategies for Optimal
Health

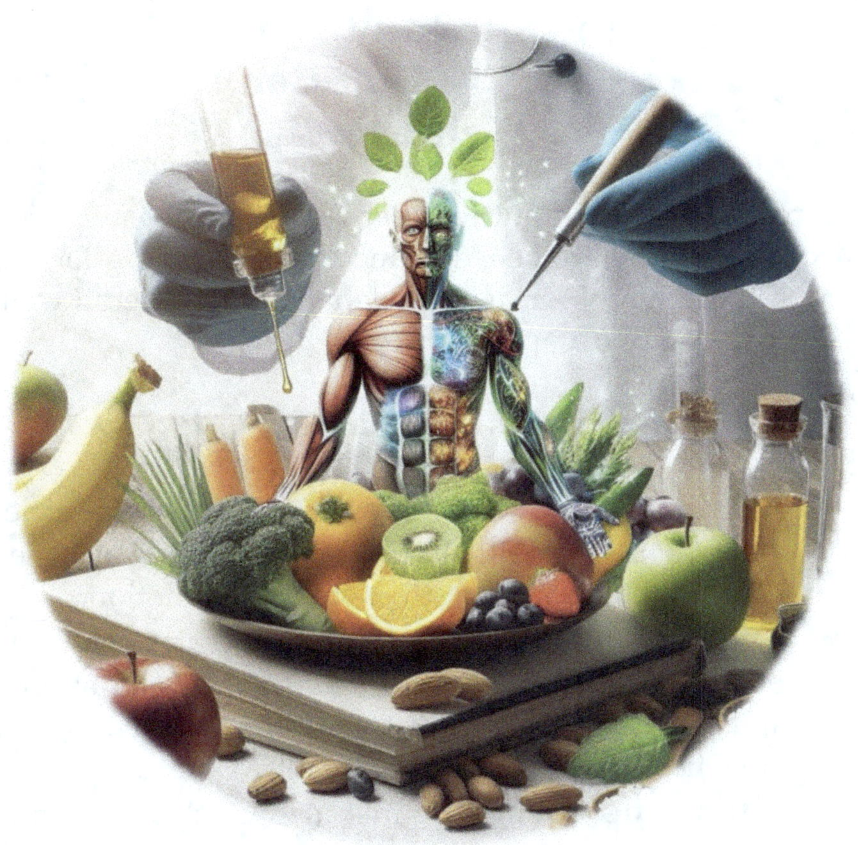

As you progress beyond the initial 30 days of your health plan, fine-tuning your nutrition can help you achieve even greater results and sustain your progress. This chapter delves into advanced nutritional strategies that can enhance your overall well-being and support your long-term health goals. By incorporating superfoods, exploring intermittent fasting, focusing on gut health, and understanding anti-inflammatory eating, you'll be equipped to take your nutrition to the next level.

Superfoods to Incorporate – Top Superfoods to Boost Nutrition and Overall Well-Being

Superfoods are nutrient-dense foods that offer exceptional health benefits. Incorporating a variety of superfoods into your diet can enhance your overall well-being and support optimal health.

Top Superfoods to Consider

- **Berries**: Blueberries, strawberries, and raspberries are rich in antioxidants, vitamins, and fiber. They help combat oxidative stress and inflammation.
- **Leafy Greens**: Spinach, kale, and Swiss chard are packed with vitamins A, C, and K, as well as iron and calcium. They support immune function and bone health.
- **Nuts and Seeds**: Almonds, chia seeds, and flaxseeds provide healthy fats, protein, and essential nutrients like omega-3 fatty acids and magnesium.

- **Quinoa**: A complete protein and a good source of fiber, quinoa contains all nine essential amino acids and supports muscle repair and energy levels.
- **Sweet Potatoes**: High in beta-carotene and vitamins A and C, sweet potatoes promote healthy vision, immune function, and skin health.

How to Incorporate Superfoods

- **Smoothies**: Blend superfoods like berries and spinach into your morning smoothie for a nutrient boost.
- **Salads**: Add nuts, seeds, and leafy greens to your salads for added crunch and nutrition.
- **Snacks**: Enjoy a handful of nuts or a serving of quinoa as a nutritious snack.

Action Step: Superfood Integration

Select a few superfoods to incorporate into your diet this week. Experiment with different recipes and meal ideas to enjoy their health benefits.

Intermittent Fasting – The Pros and Cons of Intermittent Fasting and How to Incorporate It If Desired

Intermittent fasting (IF) is an eating pattern that alternates between periods of fasting and eating. It can be an effective strategy for some people to support weight management and metabolic health.

Benefits of Intermittent Fasting

- **Weight Management**: IF can help regulate calorie intake and support fat loss by extending the fasting period between meals.
- **Metabolic Health**: It may improve insulin sensitivity and support metabolic health by allowing the body to use fat stores for energy.
- **Cellular Repair**: Fasting periods trigger cellular repair processes, such as autophagy, which may promote longevity and overall health.

Potential Drawbacks

- **Hunger and Cravings**: Some people may experience increased hunger and cravings during fasting periods, which can be challenging to manage.
- **Nutrient Intake**: There is a risk of inadequate nutrient intake if meals are not balanced and nutritious during eating windows.

Popular Intermittent Fasting Methods

- **16/8 Method**: Fast for 16 hours and eat during an 8-hour window. For example, eat between 12 PM and 8 PM.
- **5:2 Method**: Eat normally for five days of the week and restrict calories to around 500-600 on two non-consecutive days.
- **Eat-Stop-Eat**: Perform a 24-hour fast once or twice a week, such as fasting from dinner one day until dinner the next day.

Action Step: Intermittent Fasting Trial

If interested, try an intermittent fasting method for one week. Monitor how it affects your hunger, energy levels, and overall well-being. Adjust based on your experiences and preferences.

Gut Health – The Role of Probiotics, Prebiotics, and Fermented Foods in Digestive Health

Maintaining a healthy gut is essential for overall health and well-being. Probiotics, prebiotics, and fermented foods play crucial roles in supporting digestive health and a balanced microbiome.

Probiotics

- **Benefits**: Probiotics are beneficial bacteria that help maintain a healthy gut flora, support digestion, and enhance immune function.
- **Sources**: Include probiotic-rich foods such as yogurt, kefir, sauerkraut, and kimchi in your diet.

Prebiotics

- **Benefits**: Prebiotics are non-digestible fibers that feed beneficial gut bacteria, promoting their growth and activity.
- **Sources**: Consume prebiotic-rich foods like garlic, onions, bananas, and asparagus.

Fermented Foods

- **Benefits**: Fermented foods are rich in probiotics and beneficial compounds that support gut health and digestion.
- **Sources**: Add foods like kombucha, miso, and tempeh to your diet for additional probiotic benefits.

Action Step: Gut Health Enhancement

Incorporate a variety of probiotic and prebiotic foods into your meals this week. Experiment with fermented foods and observe their impact on your digestion and overall well-being.

Anti-Inflammatory Eating – How to Reduce Inflammation in the Body Through Specific Foods

Chronic inflammation is linked to various health issues, including cardiovascular disease, diabetes, and arthritis. An anti-inflammatory diet can help reduce inflammation and promote overall health.

Anti-Inflammatory Foods

- **Fruits and Vegetables**: Incorporate colorful fruits and vegetables, such as berries, cherries, spinach, and broccoli, which are rich in antioxidants and anti-inflammatory compounds.
- **Healthy Fats**: Consume omega-3 fatty acids from sources like fatty fish (salmon, mackerel), walnuts, and flaxseeds to help combat inflammation.

- **Whole Grains**: Choose whole grains like oats, brown rice, and quinoa instead of refined grains, as they have anti-inflammatory properties.
- **Herbs and Spices**: Use turmeric, ginger, and garlic in your cooking. These spices contain compounds that have been shown to reduce inflammation.

Foods to Limit

- **Processed Foods**: Reduce intake of processed foods, sugary snacks, and refined carbohydrates, which can contribute to inflammation.
- **Saturated and Trans Fats**: Minimize consumption of unhealthy fats found in fried foods, baked goods, and certain oils.

Action Step: Anti-Inflammatory Meal Plan

Create a meal plan incorporating anti-inflammatory foods and recipes. Focus on including a variety of fruits, vegetables, healthy fats, and whole grains while reducing processed and inflammatory foods.

Customizing Your Diet – How to Adjust Your Eating Plan Based on Your Individual Needs and Preferences

Personalizing your diet ensures that it aligns with your unique needs, preferences, and health goals. Customizing your eating plan can enhance adherence and effectiveness.

Factors to Consider

- **Dietary Preferences**: Take into account any dietary preferences or restrictions, such as vegetarianism, veganism, or food allergies.
- **Lifestyle and Activity Level**: Adjust your calorie and macronutrient intake based on your activity level and lifestyle. For example, active individuals may need more protein or carbohydrates.
- **Health Conditions**: Tailor your diet to address any specific health conditions or concerns, such as managing blood sugar levels or improving heart health.

Strategies for Customization

- **Consult a Professional**: Consider working with a registered dietitian or nutritionist to develop a personalized eating plan based on your individual needs.
- **Experiment and Adjust**: Experiment with different foods and meal structures to find what works best for you. Make adjustments based on how you feel and your progress towards your goals.

Action Step: Personalized Nutrition Plan

Create a customized nutrition plan that aligns with your preferences, lifestyle, and health goals. Adjust your eating plan as needed based on your experiences and progress.

The Importance of Variety – Why a Diverse Diet Is Key to Long-Term Health and How to Mix Things Up

A diverse diet is essential for obtaining a wide range of nutrients and maintaining long-term health. Eating a variety of foods ensures you receive all the necessary vitamins, minerals, and other nutrients your body needs.

Benefits of a Diverse Diet

- **Nutritional Balance**: A varied diet provides a broad spectrum of nutrients, reducing the risk of deficiencies and promoting overall health.
- **Enhanced Flavor and Enjoyment**: Trying new foods and recipes keeps meals interesting and enjoyable, which supports adherence to a healthy eating plan.
- **Reduced Risk of Chronic Diseases**: A diverse diet can help reduce the risk of chronic diseases by providing a wide range of antioxidants and phytochemicals.

Tips for Increasing Variety

- **Try New Ingredients**: Incorporate different fruits, vegetables, grains, and proteins into your meals. Explore ethnic cuisines and seasonal produce.
- **Experiment with Recipes**: Experiment with new recipes and cooking methods to keep meals exciting and varied.

- **Rotate Foods**: Avoid eating the same foods every day. Rotate your food choices to ensure a diverse nutrient intake.

Action Step: Meal Variety Plan

Develop a meal plan that includes a variety of foods and recipes. Aim to try new ingredients or dishes each week to maintain a diverse and balanced diet.

By fine-tuning your nutrition with advanced strategies, you'll enhance your overall health and well-being. Incorporate superfoods, explore intermittent fasting, focus on gut health, and practice anti-inflammatory eating to support your long-term success. Customize your diet to meet your individual needs and embrace variety to ensure a well-rounded and sustainable approach to nutrition.

Chapter 09

Building a Sustainable Lifestyle – Turning Your Plan Into Lifelong Habits

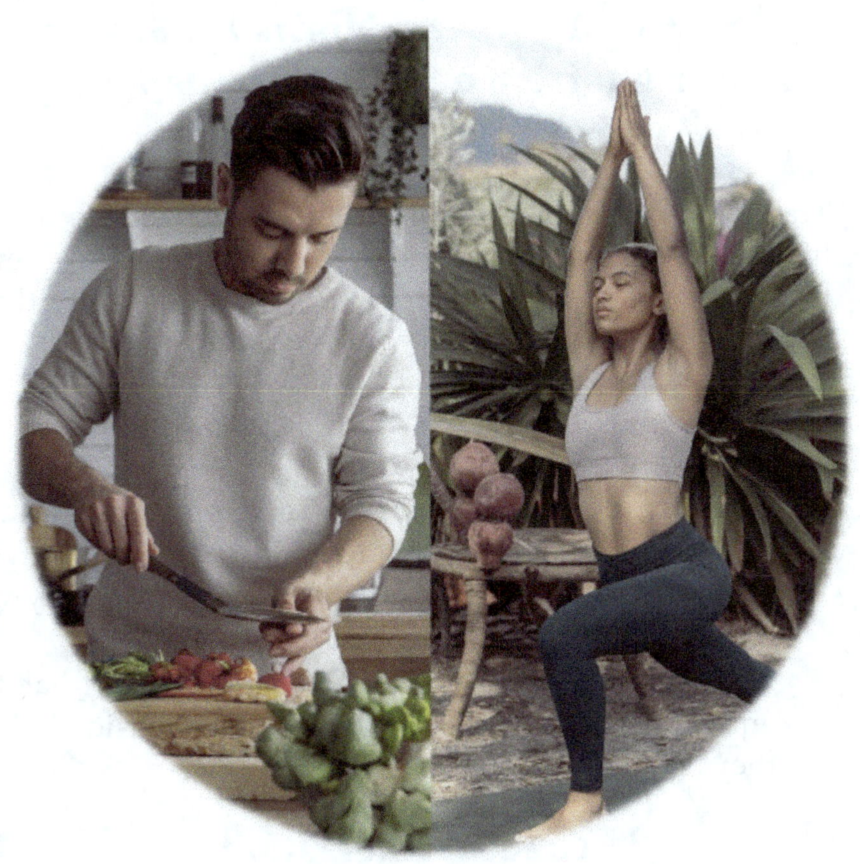

The end of your 30-day health plan marks the beginning of a new chapter in your wellness journey. To ensure that the positive changes you've made become lifelong habits, it's crucial to transition smoothly from a short-term challenge to a sustainable lifestyle. This chapter focuses on strategies to help you integrate your new habits into your everyday life, maintain motivation, and continue growing in your health journey.

Creating Your New Normal – How to Transition from a 30-Day Challenge to a Sustainable Lifestyle

Transitioning from a focused 30-day challenge to a lifelong wellness routine involves making your new habits part of your daily life. Here's how to ensure that the changes you've made become your new normal.

Reflect on Your Progress

- **Celebrate Achievements**: Take time to reflect on the progress you've made during the 30 days. Acknowledge your successes and how they've impacted your well-being.
- **Identify Key Changes**: Determine which habits and strategies worked best for you and consider how they can fit into your long-term routine.

Gradual Integration

- **Make Incremental Changes**: Gradually incorporate the habits you've developed into your daily life. Start by adding one or two new routines at a time.

- **Set Long-Term Goals**: Establish long-term health and wellness goals to keep yourself motivated and focused on continuous improvement.

Establish Routines

- **Create a Schedule**: Develop a daily or weekly schedule that includes time for meal planning, exercise, and self-care. Consistency is key to maintaining new habits.
- **Build Healthy Habits**: Integrate healthy habits into your daily routine, such as regular physical activity, balanced meals, and adequate sleep.

Action Step: New Normal Plan

Create a plan to transition your 30-day habits into your daily life. Outline specific routines and goals to maintain your progress and continue building on your success.

Meal Planning for Life – How to Make Meal Planning and Prepping a Long-Term Habit

Meal planning and prepping are essential for maintaining a healthy diet and managing your time effectively. Turning these practices into lifelong habits will help you stay on track and avoid the pitfalls of unhealthy eating.

Benefits of Meal Planning

- **Time Efficiency**: Planning and prepping meals in advance saves time during busy weekdays and reduces the likelihood of making unhealthy food choices.
- **Nutritional Control**: Meal planning allows you to control portion sizes and ensure balanced, nutritious meals.

Strategies for Effective Meal Planning

- **Weekly Planning**: Set aside time each week to plan your meals. Use a meal planner or app to organize your meals and create a shopping list.
- **Batch Cooking**: Prepare large batches of staple items such as grains, proteins, and vegetables. Store them in the fridge or freezer for easy access.
- **Prep Ingredients**: Chop vegetables, cook grains, and portion out snacks ahead of time to streamline meal preparation.

Tips for Maintaining Meal Prep

- **Involve the Family**: Get family members involved in meal planning and preparation to share the responsibility and make it more enjoyable.
- **Experiment with Recipes**: Keep meal prep interesting by trying new recipes and incorporating seasonal ingredients.

Action Step: Meal Planning Routine

Establish a weekly meal planning and prepping routine. Create a meal plan, prep ingredients, and organize your meals for the upcoming week to build consistency.

Finding Balance – How to Enjoy Indulgences Without Sabotaging Your Progress

Maintaining a healthy lifestyle doesn't mean you have to completely eliminate indulgences. Finding a balance between enjoying treats and staying on track is essential for long-term success.

The 80/20 Rule

- **Healthy Base**: Aim to eat healthily 80% of the time, focusing on nutrient-dense foods and balanced meals.
- **Flexible Indulgences**: Allow yourself to enjoy indulgent foods 20% of the time without guilt. This approach helps prevent feelings of deprivation.

Mindful Eating

- **Savor Your Treats**: When indulging, practice mindful eating by savoring each bite and paying attention to your hunger and fullness cues.
- **Portion Control**: Enjoy indulgent foods in moderation by controlling portion sizes and balancing them with healthier choices.

Planning for Indulgences

- **Plan Ahead**: If you know you'll have a special treat or event, plan your meals and snacks around it to maintain balance.
- **Healthy Alternatives**: Find healthier versions of your favorite treats or recipes to satisfy cravings while staying aligned with your goals.

Action Step: Balanced Eating Plan

Develop a plan to incorporate indulgences in a balanced way. Use the 80/20 rule and mindful eating strategies to enjoy treats while maintaining your progress.

Managing Stress and Emotional Eating – Tips for Handling Stress Without Turning to Food

Stress and emotional eating can derail your progress and impact your well-being. Learning to manage stress effectively and address emotional eating is crucial for maintaining a healthy lifestyle.

Identifying Triggers

- **Recognize Patterns**: Pay attention to situations or emotions that trigger stress or emotional eating. Keep a journal to track your triggers and responses.
- **Find Alternatives**: Develop alternative coping strategies for dealing with stress, such as exercise, meditation, or engaging in hobbies.
  - ### Stress Management Techniques

- **Mindfulness and Relaxation**: Practice mindfulness, deep breathing, or progressive muscle relaxation to manage stress and reduce its impact on your eating habits.
- **Physical Activity**: Engage in regular physical activity to release endorphins and reduce stress levels.

Emotional Eating Strategies

- **Healthy Snacks**: Keep nutritious snacks on hand to avoid turning to unhealthy options when you're emotionally driven to eat.
- **Seek Support**: Reach out to friends, family, or a therapist if you need help managing stress or emotional eating.

Action Step: Stress and Emotional Eating Plan

Create a plan to manage stress and emotional eating. Identify your triggers, implement alternative coping strategies, and seek support if needed.

Maintaining Motivation – Strategies to Keep the Momentum Going Beyond the Initial 30 Days

Staying motivated beyond the initial 30 days is key to achieving long-term success. Implementing strategies to maintain your enthusiasm and commitment will help you stay on track.

Setting New Goals

- **Short-Term Goals**: Establish new short-term goals to keep yourself motivated and focused on continuous progress.
- **Long-Term Vision**: Keep your long-term vision and aspirations in mind to maintain a sense of purpose and direction.

Tracking Progress

- **Celebrate Milestones**: Recognize and celebrate your achievements and progress. Reward yourself for reaching milestones to stay motivated.
- **Reflect Regularly**: Regularly assess your progress and adjust your goals or strategies as needed to stay on track.

Building a Support System

- **Find a Buddy**: Connect with a friend or family member who shares similar health goals for mutual support and accountability.
- **Join a Community**: Participate in online forums, support groups, or local wellness communities to stay engaged and inspired.

Action Step: Motivation Maintenance Plan

Develop a plan to maintain your motivation and commitment. Set new goals, track your progress, and build a support system to keep yourself on track.

Continuing to Learn – How to Keep Expanding Your Knowledge of Nutrition, Fitness, and Wellness

Ongoing learning and growth are essential for sustaining a healthy lifestyle. Expanding your knowledge of nutrition, fitness, and wellness will help you make informed choices and stay engaged in your health journey.

Staying Informed

- **Read Books and Articles**: Explore books, articles, and reputable websites to stay up-to-date with the latest research and trends in health and wellness.
- **Attend Workshops**: Participate in workshops, webinars, or conferences on nutrition, fitness, and wellness to gain new insights and skills.

Engaging with Experts

- **Consult Professionals**: Work with registered dietitians, fitness trainers, or wellness coaches to deepen your understanding and address specific needs.
- **Seek Guidance**: Ask questions and seek advice from experts to enhance your knowledge and make informed decisions.

Applying Knowledge

- **Experiment with New Ideas**: Test out new nutrition strategies, fitness routines, or wellness practices to see what works best for you.
- **Share What You Learn**: Share your knowledge and experiences with others to contribute to a supportive community and reinforce your own learning.

Action Step: Lifelong Learning Plan

Create a plan to continue expanding your knowledge of nutrition, fitness, and wellness. Set goals for reading, attending workshops, and engaging with experts to stay informed and motivated.

By building a sustainable lifestyle, you'll ensure that the positive changes you've made become permanent habits. Transition smoothly from the 30-day challenge, make meal planning and prepping a regular practice, and find a balance between indulgences and healthy choices. Manage stress, maintain motivation, and continue learning to support your lifelong journey to health and well-being.

Chapter 10

Celebrating Your Success –
Reflecting on Your Journey

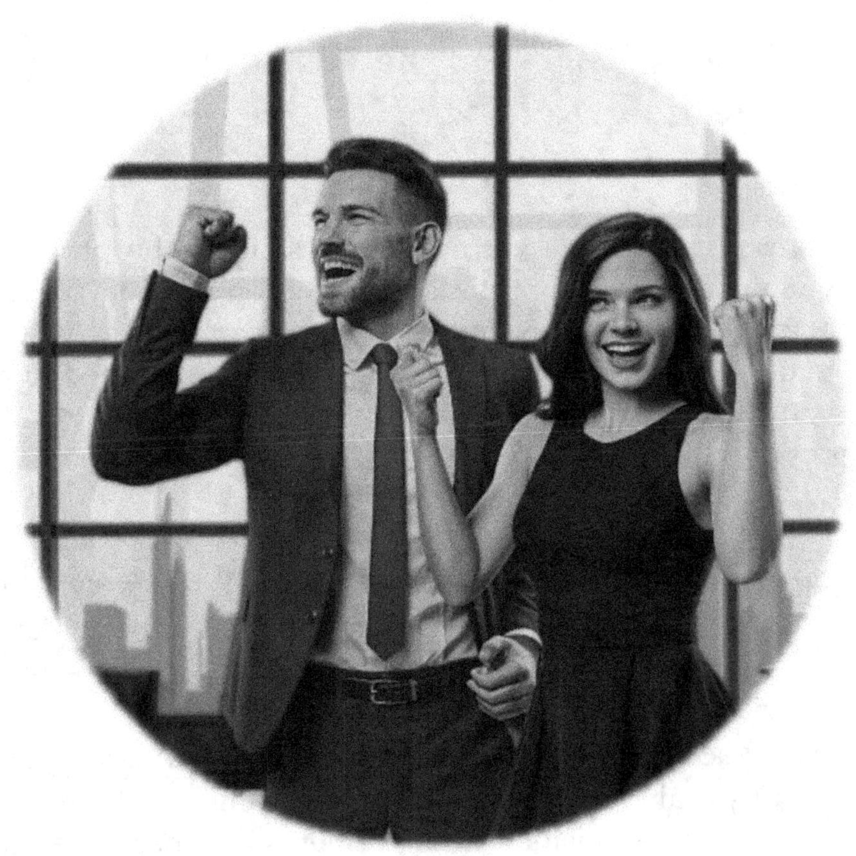

Congratulations on completing the 30-day health plan! Reaching this milestone is a significant achievement and a testament to your dedication and hard work. This final chapter is dedicated to celebrating your success, reflecting on your journey, and planning for the future. By acknowledging your progress and setting new goals, you can continue to build on your achievements and maintain a lifelong commitment to wellness.

Looking Back on the Past 30 Days – A Reflection Exercise to Recognize How Far You've Come

Reflecting on your journey helps solidify the progress you've made and provides motivation for the future. Taking time to review your accomplishments will reinforce the positive changes you've integrated into your life.

Reflection Exercise

- **Journal Your Achievements**: Write down the goals you set at the beginning of the 30 days and how you've achieved them. Include both small victories and major milestones.
- **Assess Your Progress**: Evaluate changes in your physical health, mental well-being, and overall lifestyle. Consider improvements in energy levels, mood, fitness, and dietary habits.
- **Identify Challenges Overcome**: Reflect on the obstacles you faced and how you overcame them. Recognizing your resilience will strengthen your confidence and commitment.

- **Celebrate Growth**: Acknowledge the skills and knowledge you've gained throughout the program. Appreciate how these new habits have impacted your daily life.

Action Step: Reflection Summary

Complete a reflection summary that highlights your achievements, progress, and the challenges you've overcome. Use this summary as a motivational tool and a reminder of your hard work.

What's Next? – How to Set New Health Goals That Build on Your 30-Day Success

Building on your 30-day success involves setting new health goals that continue to challenge and inspire you. Creating a roadmap for the future will help you maintain momentum and stay focused on your long-term wellness journey.

Setting New Goals

- **Review Your Progress**: Consider your reflection summary and identify areas where you'd like to continue growing or improving.
- **Establish SMART Goals**: Set Specific, Measurable, Achievable, Relevant, and Time-bound goals to ensure they are clear and attainable. For example, aim to increase your weekly exercise duration or incorporate a new healthy food into your diet.

- **Create a Plan**: Develop a detailed action plan for achieving your new goals. Break down the steps required and set a timeline for reaching them.

Example Goals

- **Fitness Goal**: Increase your weekly workout sessions from three to five, incorporating different types of exercise such as strength training and cardio.
- **Nutrition Goal**: Add two new vegetables to your meals each week to diversify your nutrient intake.
- **Wellness Goal**: Implement a daily mindfulness practice, such as meditation or yoga, to enhance mental well-being.

Action Step: New Goal Setting

Set at least three new health goals that build on your 30-day success. Create an actionable plan with specific steps and deadlines to achieve these goals.

Rewarding Yourself – Non-Food-Related Ways to Celebrate Your Progress

Celebrating your achievements is an important part of maintaining motivation and reinforcing positive behavior. Choose rewards that honor your progress without involving food.

Non-Food-Related Rewards

- **Pamper Yourself**: Treat yourself to a spa day, massage, or relaxing bath to celebrate your hard work.
- **Get Active**: Purchase new workout gear, a fitness tracker, or a membership to a fitness class you've been wanting to try.
- **Enjoy Experiences**: Plan a fun outing, such as a hike, a cultural event, or a day trip to celebrate your achievements.
- **Personal Treats**: Invest in something meaningful, like a book you've been wanting to read or a new hobby-related item.

Action Step: Reward Plan

Choose at least two non-food-related rewards to celebrate your progress. Plan how and when you will treat yourself to these rewards as a way to acknowledge your success.

Sharing Your Journey – The Power of Inspiring Others and Building a Health-Conscious Community

Sharing your journey not only allows you to celebrate your achievements but also inspires and motivates others. Building a community of like-minded individuals can enhance your support network and promote collective wellness.

Ways to Share Your Journey

- **Social Media**: Share your progress and insights on social media platforms to inspire your network and connect with others on similar health journeys.
- **Support Groups**: Join or create a local or online support group where you can share experiences, offer encouragement, and exchange tips with others.
- **Blogging or Vlogging**: Start a blog or YouTube channel to document your journey, share your successes and challenges, and provide valuable advice to others.

Benefits of Sharing

- **Inspiration**: Your story can motivate others to embark on their own health journeys and make positive changes in their lives.
- **Community Building**: Connecting with others who share your health goals fosters a sense of community and mutual support.

Action Step: Share Your Story

Decide how you will share your journey with others. Whether through social media, support groups, or a personal blog, take the steps to inspire and connect with those around you.

Tracking Long-Term Success – Tools and Strategies for Measuring Progress Over Time

Long-term success requires ongoing monitoring and evaluation of your progress. Using tools and strategies to track your achievements will help you stay accountable and make necessary adjustments.

Tools for Tracking

- **Health Apps**: Use health and wellness apps to track your nutrition, exercise, and overall progress. Many apps offer features like goal setting, progress charts, and reminders.
- **Journals**: Maintain a health journal to record your daily activities, meals, and reflections. Regular journaling helps you stay aware of your habits and progress.
- **Regular Assessments**: Schedule periodic assessments to review your progress, such as monthly fitness tests, nutrition reviews, or wellness check-ins.

Strategies for Tracking

- **Set Milestones**: Define key milestones to achieve throughout the year and track your progress towards them.
- **Adjust Goals**: Regularly review and adjust your goals based on your progress and any changes in your health or lifestyle.

Action Step: Tracking Plan

Develop a tracking plan that includes tools and strategies for monitoring your long-term success. Set up regular check-ins to evaluate your progress and make adjustments as needed.

Staying Committed to Lifelong Wellness – How to Stay Focused on Health for the Rest of Your Life

Maintaining a lifelong commitment to wellness involves integrating healthy habits into your daily life and continuously pursuing personal growth. By staying focused and adapting to changes, you can sustain your health achievements for the long term.

Key Principles for Lifelong Wellness

- **Consistency**: Prioritize consistency in your healthy habits, even when faced with challenges or changes in your routine.
- **Adaptability**: Be flexible and adapt your wellness plan as needed to accommodate life changes, such as new responsibilities or health conditions.
- **Self-Care**: Continue to prioritize self-care practices that support your physical, mental, and emotional well-being.

Ongoing Growth

- **Set New Challenges**: Regularly challenge yourself with new health and wellness goals to keep your journey engaging and rewarding.
- **Stay Educated**: Keep learning about nutrition, fitness, and wellness to stay informed and inspired.

Action Step: Lifelong Commitment Plan

Create a plan to stay committed to lifelong wellness. Include principles for consistency, adaptability, and self-care, and outline strategies for ongoing growth and education.

Celebrating your success and reflecting on your journey is an essential part of maintaining a healthy lifestyle. By setting new goals, rewarding yourself, sharing your journey, and tracking long-term success, you'll continue to build on your achievements and stay focused on your lifelong commitment to wellness. Embrace this next phase of your journey with enthusiasm and confidence, knowing that you have the tools and strategies to support your ongoing health and well-being.

Conclusion

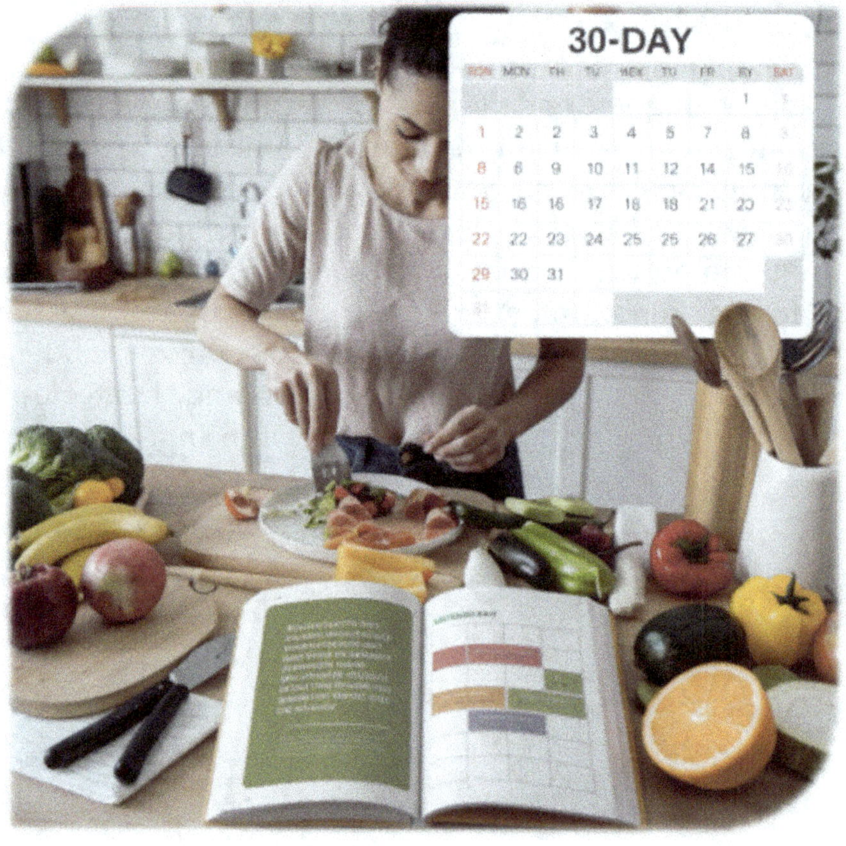

Your Health Journey Never Ends

As you conclude this 30-day health plan, it's essential to recognize that your journey toward wellness is a lifelong endeavor. This final chapter serves as a reminder that achieving and maintaining health is not a destination but an ongoing process. Embracing this journey with a positive mindset and a commitment to continual growth will set the foundation for a fulfilling and balanced life.

A Lifetime Commitment – Embracing Health as a Long-Term Journey Rather Than a Short-Term Challenge

Your commitment to health extends far beyond the initial 30 days. Embracing this journey as a lifelong pursuit allows you to integrate healthy habits into your daily life and make wellness a core aspect of who you are.

Long-Term Perspective

- **Health as a Lifestyle**: View health not as a series of short-term goals but as a lifestyle that you cultivate and maintain. This perspective encourages sustainable changes rather than temporary fixes.
- **Ongoing Growth**: Recognize that health is an evolving journey with opportunities for growth and improvement at every stage. Embrace each step as part of your ongoing development.

Building a Supportive Environment

- **Create Healthy Habits**: Continue to build and reinforce healthy habits that align with your long-term goals. These habits will become integral parts of your daily routine.
- **Surround Yourself with Support**: Cultivate a supportive environment by connecting with friends, family, or communities that share your wellness values and goals.

Action Step: Long-Term Health Plan

Develop a plan to integrate wellness into your long-term lifestyle. Outline specific habits and practices that you will maintain and adapt as part of your daily routine.

Embracing Imperfection – Why Setbacks Are Normal and How to Keep Moving Forward After Slip-Ups

Setbacks are a natural part of any journey, and it's crucial to approach them with understanding and resilience. Embracing imperfection helps you navigate challenges without losing sight of your overall goals.

Accepting Setbacks

- **Normalize Imperfection**: Understand that setbacks and challenges are a normal part of the process. Everyone experiences them, and they do not define your success.
- **Learn and Adapt**: Use setbacks as opportunities to learn and adapt. Reflect on what went wrong,

adjust your strategies, and continue moving forward with renewed determination.

Strategies for Moving Forward

- **Self-Compassion**: Practice self-compassion by treating yourself with kindness and understanding. Avoid self-criticism and focus on constructive solutions.
- **Revisit Goals**: Reassess your goals and strategies as needed to address any obstacles you encounter. Adjust your plan to better align with your current needs and circumstances.

Action Step: Setback Management Plan

Create a plan for handling setbacks and challenges. Include strategies for maintaining a positive mindset, learning from experiences, and adjusting your goals as needed.

Finding Joy in the Process – How to Maintain a Positive Relationship with Food, Fitness, and Your Body

Maintaining a positive relationship with food, fitness, and your body is key to enjoying the journey and achieving long-term success. Finding joy in the process ensures that your wellness journey is fulfilling and sustainable.

Joyful Approach

- **Positive Mindset**: Focus on the positive aspects of your health journey, such as increased energy, improved mood, and enhanced well-being. Celebrate the small victories and progress you make.
- **Enjoy the Process**: Find pleasure in the activities that contribute to your health, such as trying new recipes, exploring different forms of exercise, or practicing self-care.

Body Appreciation

- **Practice Gratitude**: Cultivate gratitude for your body and its capabilities. Appreciate the strength, resilience, and health that you have.
- **Avoid Comparisons**: Focus on your own journey and progress rather than comparing yourself to others. Embrace your unique path to wellness.

Action Step: Joyful Wellness Plan

Develop a plan to incorporate joy and positivity into your wellness journey. Include practices that enhance your enjoyment of food, fitness, and body appreciation.

Becoming Your Best Self – Reflecting on How the Changes You've Made Impact Not Just Your Body, but Your Mind and Life

The changes you've made during this 30-day health plan have likely impacted more than just your physical health. Reflect on how these changes have influenced your overall well-being and personal growth.

Holistic Impact

- **Mind and Body Connection**: Recognize how improvements in your physical health have positively affected your mental and emotional well-being.
- **Enhanced Quality of Life**: Reflect on how adopting a healthier lifestyle has contributed to a more fulfilling and balanced life, including better relationships, increased self-esteem, and greater life satisfaction.

Personal Growth

- **Self-Discovery**: Appreciate the personal growth and self-discovery that has occurred as a result of your commitment to health and wellness.
- **New Perspectives**: Embrace the new perspectives and insights you've gained about yourself and your capabilities.

Action Step: Reflective Growth Plan

Create a plan to continue reflecting on and celebrating the impact of your health journey. Include practices for recognizing personal growth and acknowledging the positive changes in your life.

Keep Evolving – A Reminder to Stay Curious, Keep Learning, and Always Strive for Improvement

The pursuit of health and wellness is an ongoing journey of curiosity and growth. Staying curious and committed to learning ensures that you continue to evolve and enhance your well-being.

Lifelong Learning

- **Explore New Areas**: Stay open to exploring new aspects of health and wellness, such as emerging nutrition trends, innovative fitness routines, or holistic practices.
- **Seek Knowledge**: Engage in continuous learning through books, courses, workshops, or consultations with health professionals to deepen your understanding and stay motivated.

Embrace Change

- **Adapt and Evolve**: Be willing to adapt your wellness plan as your needs and circumstances change. Embrace new challenges and opportunities for growth.
- **Celebrate Progress**: Regularly celebrate your achievements and progress, no matter how small. Use these celebrations as motivation to continue evolving.

Action Step: Evolution Plan

Develop a plan for continuous learning and evolution in your health journey. Set goals for exploring new areas of interest, seeking knowledge, and embracing change.

Your health journey is a lifelong endeavor that requires dedication, adaptability, and a positive mindset. By embracing health as a continuous process, accepting setbacks, finding joy in the journey, reflecting on your growth, and staying curious, you'll maintain a fulfilling and balanced approach to wellness. Celebrate your success, cherish the progress you've made, and look forward to the endless opportunities for growth and improvement that lie ahead. Your commitment to lifelong wellness will lead to a healthier, happier, and more vibrant life.